SWISS BALL
CORE WORKOUT

Declan Condron

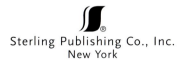

Sterling Publishing Co., Inc.
New York

Library of Congress Cataloging-in-Publication Data

Condron, Declan.
    Swiss ball core workout / Declan Condron.
        p. cm.
    Includes index.
    ISBN-13: 978-1-4027-4214-9
    ISBN-10: 1-4027-4214-2
1. Swiss exercise balls. 2. Exercise. I. Title.

GV484.C66 2006
613.7'10284--dc22

2006025309

2 4 6 8 10 9 7 5 3 1

Published by Sterling Publishing Co., Inc.
387 Park Avenue South, New York, NY 10016
© 2006 by PumpOne
Distributed in Canada by Sterling Publishing
c/o Canadian Manda Group, 165 Dufferin Street
Toronto, Ontario, Canada M6K 3H6
Distributed in the United Kingdom by GMC Distribution Services
Castle Place, 166 High Street, Lewes, East Sussex, England BN7 1XU
Distributed in Australia by Capricorn Link (Australia) Pty. Ltd.
P.O. Box 704, Windsor, NSW 2756, Australia

Photographs by Craig Schlossberg / PumpOne

Book design by Judith Stagnitto Abbate / Abbate Design

Sterling ISBN-13: 978-1-4027-4214-9
ISBN-10: 1-4027-4214-2

For information about custom editions, special sales, premium and
corporate purchases, please contact Sterling Special Sales
Department at 800-805-5489 or specialsales@sterlingpub.com.

Contents

(W) ELCOME TO the *Swiss Ball Core Workout.* This book is designed to provide multiple workouts using a Swiss ball, some light dumbbells, ankle weights, and a mat. These workouts can be done anywhere: at home, while traveling, or at the gym (most gyms will have all the equipment).

Using a Swiss ball for exercising is not a new concept. The ball has been used for rehabilitation and physical therapy for many years. It was first introduced in Switzerland in 1963, earning the name Swiss ball. (It's sometimes called a gymnastic ball, or a fit ball.) Swiss balls gained popularity in gyms and health clubs in the 1990s and are now standard equipment in most exercise facilities.

This book on Swiss ball core training is not just a list of exercises but provides specific, graduated workouts. Workouts are divided into three levels with four or five workouts each, with each level progressively more challenging. This book will guide you on the proper form for each exercise as it takes you through the three levels of structured workouts.

SO WHAT'S THE BIG DEAL WITH THE BALL?

Why use a Swiss ball? It looks slippery and unstable. Might be a little dangerous? What can it do for you? Swiss balls are completely safe and offer many benefits for fitness training. Actually, it's the very instability of a Swiss ball that makes it such an excellent exercise tool. Just by sitting on the ball, you activate the stabilizer muscles of your core.

SOME BENEFITS:

Increased neuromuscular functioning

The neuromuscular system is the connection between the brain, central nervous system, and the muscles. To perform a movement or action, your brain sends a message via the nervous system to the muscles to go into action. Using a Swiss ball involves greater muscle activity and ignites more and better-quality messages moving through the nerve-muscle conduit from the brain.

Improvements in coordination and proprioception

As the brain communicates with the muscles, the muscles talk back to the brain. This is called proprioception, and sometimes kinesthesia. Muscles sense where your limbs are in space and signal your brain: "Your left arm is above your head," or "Your right leg is straight out in front." A Swiss ball challenges proprioception because it is less stable than a bench and requires quick adjustment to maintain balance. This messaging between the brain and muscles builds better coordination and proprioception.

Develop better muscle synergy

Contrary to popular belief, a muscle group does not work by itself. Muscle groups work together to facilitate movement, and also to stabilize and support inert body parts. For example, during a biceps curl, your biceps muscles contract to move your arm, while your deltoid muscles help the movement and also stabilize your shoulder. Meanwhile, the triceps work to control the speed of the movement. Using a Swiss ball can help develop better synergy between muscle groups.

Variety

Our bodies are very smart machines. When our brain asks us to move, the brain figures out the easiest way to do it. Asked to perform a movement again and again, it becomes increasingly easy. Changing the task slightly gives our bodies a new challenge: to figure out a better way to meet new requirements. A Swiss ball is a great tool to change a workout and give the body new stimuli.

The Core Defined

OUR BODY'S CORE is defined as the deep abdominal and spinal muscles that support the spine and help to maintain a neutral position during movement. This is just partly true. The definition of the core can be expanded to include almost all the muscles of the torso. This includes the smaller deep muscles, such as the *transverse abdominus* and *multifidus*, but also the larger muscles such as the *rectus abdominus*, *quadratus lumborum* (lower back muscles that maintain spinal and pelvic balance), internal and external obliques, the *erector spinae*, the *latissimus dorsi* and *iliopsoas* muscles.

This muscular core acts like a corset that can stabilize, move, resist movement, and lend support all at once. Remember, muscle groups don't act in isolation; they act in synergy to produce the best movement strategy possible. Therefore, core muscles work together to produce the most efficient movement, not always the safest movement.

THE SWISS BALL AND THE BACK

Back pain is one of the most common physical problems in the U.S. today. It is estimated that eight out of ten people will suffer some form of back pain in their life. These statistics are not very encouraging, but there is hope: With good overall fitness, we can greatly reduce this risk. Originally, the Swiss ball was used to rehabilitate adults with orthopedic injuries, including back injuries. Any of us can go a long way in keeping our backs strong, healthy, and free of injury by using a Swiss ball to strengthen core muscle groups.

A WORD ABOUT POSTURE

Posture can be defined as the position or bearing of the body. It refers to the overall alignment of body parts to each other when standing in a relaxed position. Posture is the result of many processes and tensions in the body. It becomes a measure of overall balance. Poor posture can lead to mechanical problems, dysfunctions, and pain.

Let's take a look at the spine. If a person can position his spine so his vertebrae are aligned over one another without lateral curvature, and his muscles, ligaments, and tendons balance his weight with minimal effort, he is in a good neutral spinal posture with respect to the force of gravity. If, however, one vertebra is off track, or one muscle is not functioning, alignment is off, and can cause excessive stress on the spine, resulting in injury.

Exercise, stretching, and massage can help to restore balance and good posture. A Swiss ball is an excellent training stimulus. In these workouts, you will see the phrase "maintain a neutral spine." This refers to having good posture throughout the spine.

A S WITH ANY EXERCISE PROGRAM, safety is of the utmost importance. The last thing you want to do is to injure yourself trying to get into better shape and improve your health. Before you start, we recommend you do the following:

TALK TO YOUR DOCTOR

Always consult your doctor before starting a fitness program, especially if you have or have had a chronic medical condition, are taking any medications, or are pregnant.

Immediately stop exercising if you feel pain, faintness, dizziness, or shortness of breath. Wait awhile. You may decide to quit for the day, or resume slowly.

GET EQUIPPED

Check the condition of the Swiss ball and any other equipment. Make sure you choose the right ball for your body size. Follow the manufacturer's instructions for inflation, and read all warnings and instructions on the proper use and maintenance of all equipment.

MAKE ROOM AND SUIT UP

Make sure you have enough space to exercise, and avoid exercising on slippery surfaces. Be aware of the surrounding areas, other people, and any obstacles that might cause a fall.

Wear appropriate exercise clothing that is neither too baggy nor too tight. Also be sure to wear some form of footwear. Sneakers are comfortable and have a nonslip sole.

WARM UP AND COOL DOWN

Always warm up for at least five minutes before starting any workout. Warming up gets the body ready to exercise and increases its core temperature and muscle elasticity. We have provided some warm up tips a little later in the book.

Also be sure to cool down and stretch after your workout. This will help relax your muscles and return them to their resting length, and reduce to normal your core temperature. We have included a number of specific stretches to do after each workout.

HAVE WATER ON HAND

It's a good idea to eat something at least two hours before exercising, and always to have water on hand while you are working out. Right after working out is a great time to replenish the body's energy supplies, while you relax and rest.

Equipment

T HE WORKOUTS IN THIS BOOK require the use of the following equipment:

1. SWISS BALL

It wouldn't be much of a Swiss ball exercise program without a Swiss ball. They come in various sizes and colors. Be sure to choose the correct ball for you. Manufacturers provide size guidelines based on height. A general rule of thumb is that when seated on the ball, your hips should be slightly higher than your knees, and your feet should be flat on the floor.

The following size chart can be used as a general rule.

Ball Size Guidelines for Exercise

HEIGHT	BALL SIZE
Under 5'2" (*1.57 m*)	45 cm
5'3"– 5'8" (*1.60 m–1.72 m*)	55 cm
5'9"– 6'2" (*1.75 m–1.88 m*)	65 cm
Above 6'3" (*1.90 m*)	75 cm

Inflate the ball according to the manufacturers' guidelines. Most balls come with a hand or foot pump.

2. DUMBBELLS

Weighted dumbbells come in many shapes and sizes and many appealing colors. Since you will be using different muscle groups, some bigger and stronger than others, we recommend having a selection of sizes. A range from 5–15 pounds should be sufficient at first. You can always add more weight as you gain strength and tone your muscles.

3. ANKLE WEIGHTS

Ankle weights are great for adding resistance to exercises for the lower limbs. We recommend the wraparound type with adjustable weight inserts, easily removed or replaced when necessary.

4. EXERCISE MAT

Some of our exercises require you to lie on the floor. It's a good idea to work on a basic yoga or pilates mat. The mat will also provide a nonslip surface during other exercises.

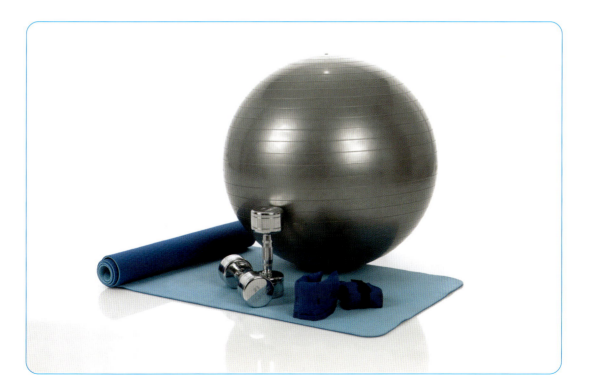

How This Book Works

THIS BOOK IS ORGANIZED to provide a progressive exercise plan. Like a personal trainer, it is a guide to what exercises to perform, in which order, and when to advance to a new level to keep you working toward a stronger, fitter body.

The book is divided into three difficulty levels, each containing four or five workouts. Every workout contains from eight to fifteen different exercises that vary in time from 25 to 55 minutes. The side-tab color stays the same for all the exercises within each workout in a particular level for easy color reference to the workouts.

Workouts can be performed at different intensities by varying the number of repetitions and sets, the load used, and the amount of rest between sets. The book offers two different intensity tracks for each workout: the **toning track** and the **weight-loss track**. The **toning track** concentrates on building strength and defining muscles; the **weight-loss track** concentrates on losing weight. There is some cross-over between tracks: If you are on the **weight-loss track**, you will also see increases in muscle strength and definition; on the **toning track**, you might also lose weight.

We suggest beginning at level one and working your way up to level three, even if you are already experienced with workouts. Level three workouts can be very challenging and may take some time to master, so take your time and enjoy the journey. Whether you choose the **toning** or **weight-loss track**, try to do two-to-three workout sessions per week. Just as the body needs variety, it also needs consistency. Perform each workout a few times in each level before moving forward. Spend a number of weeks rotating through the workouts in level one before attempting levels two and three.

A PLAN FOR TOTAL HEALTH

Exercising with a Swiss ball should be part of a plan for total health, a plan that takes some dedication and hard work. No one gets fit and strong overnight. An overall health plan should incorporate a number of practices and habits that have an impact on your body. There are five essential components to a health plan: strength training; cardiovascular training; flexibility and mobility; a healthy nutrition plan; and adequate rest and recovery. An effective Swiss ball exercise program depends on all five of these measures. The right emphasis on each depends on your individual goal.

I F THIS IS YOUR FIRST TIME using a Swiss ball, or if it's been a while, take some time to get familiar with balancing on the ball. Practice the three positions below, and once you are comfortable, you are ready to start working out. Do not hold your breath; whether you breathe in or out as you lift the dumbbells is not as important as remembering to breath.

SIT ON THE BALL

Sit on the top center of the ball with your feet flat on the floor. Your hips should be slightly higher than your knees. Keep your head up and look straight ahead, aligning your shoulders over your hips. Be conscious of the position of your spine at all times. Do not let your shoulders roll forward, or flex your lower back. This will help you establish good posture along your spine while seated on the ball.

LIE ON THE BALL

Lie face down with the ball under your midsection and your hands and feet on the floor. Practice rolling forward and backward, lifting your hands or feet as you roll. When you feel comfortable with these movements, move side to side. Work up to lying on the ball without your hands or feet touching the floor.

Next, turn over on your back and center the ball between your shoulder blades. Place your feet flat on the floor and your hands on your hips. Keep your hips level with your shoulders while contracting your abdominal and core muscles. This is known as the reverse bridge position.

KNEEL ON THE BALL

For this position, keep something sturdy like a chair or bench close by to help with balance. Place both hands and one knee on top of the ball. Slowly lift your other leg off the floor, and place on the ball. You should now be on all fours atop the ball. Now place one hand on the chair to help stabilize you, and lift the other hand off the ball. Move your upper body upright. Be conscious of the position of your spine; do not let your shoulders roll forward or flex your lower back. Take your hand off the support and practice holding your body upright. You will move around some, so try to find your center of balance.

Tips for Warming Up and Cooling Down

A WARM-UP IS A CRUCIAL PART of any exercise program. The importance of a structured warm-up can not be overstated. It is essential for getting the body ready for activity and helping prevent injury. Warming up before working out prepares you for strenuous activity by increasing the temperatures of both the body's core and muscles. Increasing muscle temperature helps to loosen them, making them more supple and flexible.

Warming up also increases your heart rate and the rate of your blood flow to your muscles, increasing the delivery of oxygen and nutrients to them and helping prepare them and other tissues for activity.

A concise warm-up should last 10 to 15 minutes. It should target all areas of the body, starting with gentle activity such as light cardiovascular work. It should gradually increase in intensity, building up to movements similar to the exercises in the workout. Static stretching before working out is optional.

Just as important as warming-up before exercising is a good cooldown afterwards. Cooling down helps return your core temperature to normal and helps muscles relax and return to their original length. Static stretching during a cooldown can help to increase muscle and joint range of motion, which will improve flexibility and may reduce muscle soreness. Five specific stretches at the end of each workout will target the major muscle groups that have been used.

SQUAT TO BALL OVERHEAD

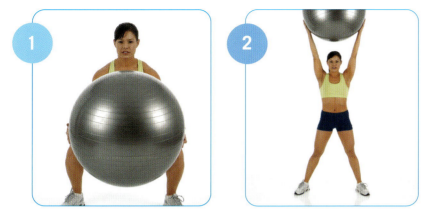

- Start in a squat position with your feet flat and your back in a neutral position. Hold the ball out in front of you at waist height.
- Stand tall and raise the ball overhead, extending your arms fully.
- Perform 10 to 15 repetitions. Be sure to squat as low as you can and to stretch as high as you can.

OVERHEAD CIRCLES

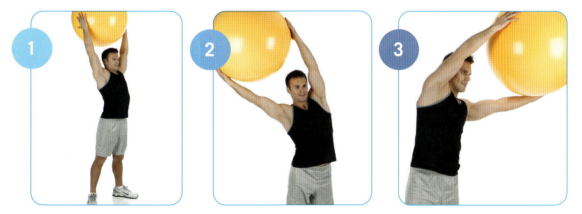

- Hold the ball overhead with your arms fully extended. Make a big circle overhead with the ball, moving through your midsection.
- Repeat the movement in the opposite direction.
- Perform 10 to 15 repetitions in each direction.

SIDE ROTATIONS

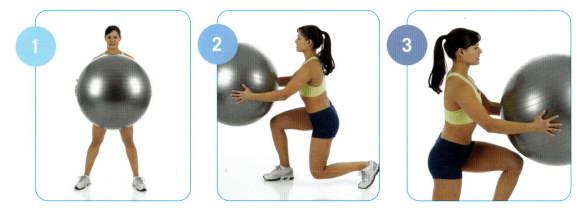

- Stand upright, holding the ball at waist height. Rotate to one side, bending your hips and knees, and lowering your body toward the floor. Switch sides, holding the ball at waist height throughout.
- Keep your head up and look straight ahead to maintain a neutral spine. Perform 10 to 15 repetitions in both directions.

SEATED TRUNK ROTATIONS

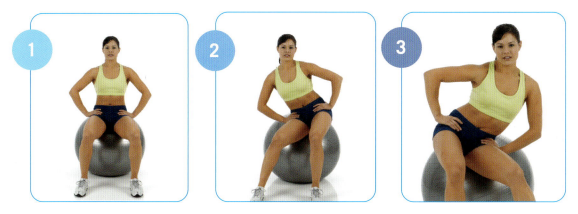

- Sit upright on the ball with your hands on your hips. Rotate your midsection, making a big circle while still seated.
- Repeat the movement in the opposite direction.
- Perform 10 to 15 repetitions in both directions.

Workout 1: WALL SQUAT

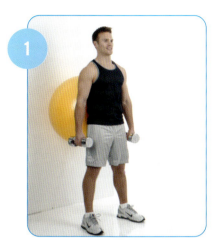

1

- Start with the ball against the wall at the level of your lower back.

- Place your feet ahead of the ball, hip-width apart with your legs straight.

- Hold a dumbbell in each hand.

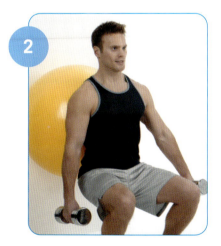

2

- Lower your body toward the floor, pushing back slightly against the ball.

- Stop when your thighs are parallel to the floor.

- Push through your feet to return to your starting position.

Intensity

Weight Loss	Toning
2 SETS	3 SETS
20 REPS	12 REPS
30-SECOND REST	30-SECOND REST
BETWEEN SETS	BETWEEN SETS

HINTS

Keep your head up and look straight ahead. Do not look down at the floor or your feet. • *Keep your feet flat on the floor as you move up and down.* • *Keep pushing back against the ball throughout the exercise.*

WORKOUT 1: Chest Press

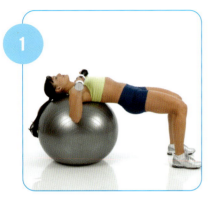

- Lie with the ball under your shoulders in a reverse bridge position. The ball should be centered between your shoulder blades.
- Keep your hips level with your shoulders and your feet flat on the floor.
- Keep your stomach muscles tight.
- Hold a dumbbell in each hand at shoulder level.

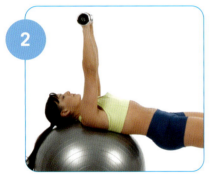

- Lift the dumbbells until your arms are straight, and the dumbbells are directly over your upper chest.
- Slowly lower the dumbbells by bending your elbows.
- Be sure to lower the dumbbells back to your shoulder level.

Intensity

Weight Loss	*Toning*
2 SETS	3 SETS
20 REPS	12 REPS
30-SECOND REST	30-SECOND REST
BETWEEN SETS	BETWEEN SETS

HINTS

Keep your hips in line with your shoulders by contracting your abdominal and core muscles. • Hold the dumbbells directly over your chest. • Start with your feet shoulder-width apart. Move your feet closer together to challenge your stability.

WORKOUT 1: Close Grip Row

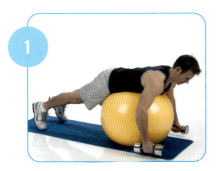

- Lie facedown with the ball under your mid-abdomen and your legs stretched out behind.

- Hold a dumbbell in each hand with your arms extended at the sides and your elbows slightly bent with palms facing each other.

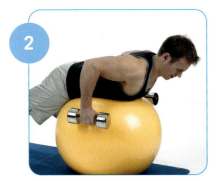

- Lift the dumbbells by drawing your shoulder blades together and bending your elbows.

- Lower the dumbbells back toward the floor to the starting position, extending at the elbows.

Intensity

Weight Loss	Toning
2 SETS	3 SETS
20 REPS	12 REPS
30-SECOND REST	30-SECOND REST
BETWEEN SETS	BETWEEN SETS

HINTS

Start with your feet shoulder-width apart. To increase the challenge to your stability, move your feet closer together. • Draw your elbows up by your sides, not outward. • Look down at the floor to keep your head in line with your spine. • Hold your head steady as you raise the dumbbells.

WORKOUT 1: Seated Overhead Press

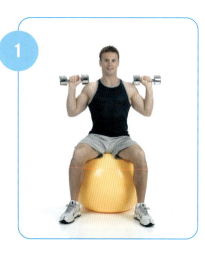

- Sit upright on the ball with your feet flat on the floor.

- Hold a dumbbell in each hand at shoulder level with your palms facing out.

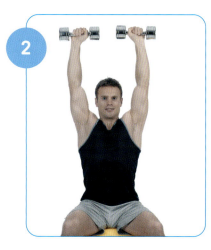

- Press the dumbbells straight overhead extending your arms.

- Lower the dumbbells by bending your elbows to return to the starting position.

- Be sure to go all the way down until the dumbbells are at your shoulder level.

Intensity

Weight Loss	Toning
2 SETS	3 SETS
20 REPS	12 REPS
30-SECOND REST	30-SECOND REST
BETWEEN SETS	BETWEEN SETS

HINTS

Keep your back upright by contracting your core muscles as you push the dumbbells overhead. • Do not round your lower back. • Complete the full range of motion, from shoulder level, to arms fully extended overhead, and back again. • Start with your feet shoulder-width apart. To increase the challenge to your stability, move your feet closer together.

WORKOUT 1: Seated Straight Biceps Curl

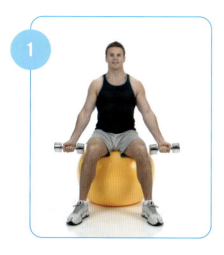

- Sit upright on the ball with your feet shoulder-width apart and flat on the floor.

- Hold a dumbbell in each hand with your palms facing forward and your arms extended by your sides.

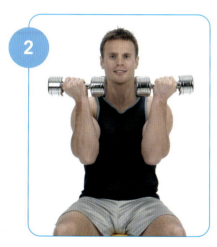

- Slowly raise the dumbbells in front to shoulder level, bending your elbows.

- Lower the dumbbells slowly, straightening your elbows to return to the starting position.

- Be sure to lower the dumbbells until your arms are fully extended.

Intensity

Weight Loss	Toning
2 SETS	3 SETS
20 REPS	12 REPS
30-SECOND REST	30-SECOND REST
BETWEEN SETS	BETWEEN SETS

HINTS

The instability of the Swiss ball adds a balance aspect to this simple exercise. • Keep your back upright by contracting your core muscles. Do not round your lower back. • Complete the full range of motion, from arms fully extended, to dumbbells at shoulder level, and back again. • Start with your feet about shoulder-width apart. To increase the challenge to your stability, move your feet closer together.

WORKOUT 1: Single-Arm Triceps Extension

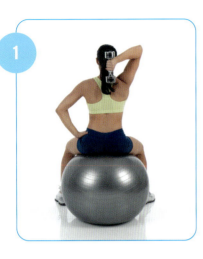

- Sit upright on the ball with your feet flat on the floor.
- Hold a dumbbell in one hand behind your head with your elbow bent and pointing up.

- Lift the dumbbell, by extending your elbow and straightening your arm directly overhead.
- Lower the dumbbell by bending your elbow, returning to the starting position behind your head.

Intensity

Weight Loss	Toning
2 SETS	3 SETS
20 REPS	12 REPS
30-SECOND REST	30-SECOND REST
BETWEEN SETS	BETWEEN SETS

HINTS

Keep your back upright by contracting your core muscles. Do not round your lower back. • Be careful not to hit the back of your head as you lift and lower the dumbbell. • Complete the full range of motion, from behind your head to having your arm fully extended overhead, and back again. • Keep your shoulder steady. Do not allow your upper arm to move around; all movement should occur at the elbow joint.

WORKOUT 1: Crunch with Feet on Ball

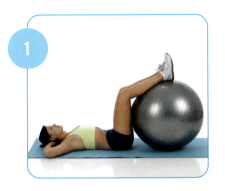

- Lie flat on your back on the mat, knees bent, with your heels on top of the ball.
- Place your hands at the sides of your head.

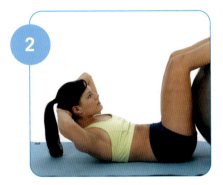

- Lift your head and shoulders off the mat while contracting your abdominals.
- Slowly roll your head and shoulders back to the mat, returning to the starting position.

Intensity

Weight Loss	Toning
2 SETS	3 SETS
20 REPS	12 REPS
30-SECOND REST	30-SECOND REST
BETWEEN SETS	BETWEEN SETS

HINTS

Make an effort to control the movement through your midsection, and avoid jerky movements. • *Don't use your hands to pull up your head and neck.* • *Raise only your head and shoulders.*

WORKOUT 1: Kneeling Oblique Crunch

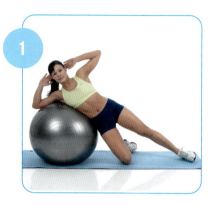

- Lie on one side on the ball with one knee on the mat and the other leg stretched out to the side.

- Place your hands at the sides of your head.

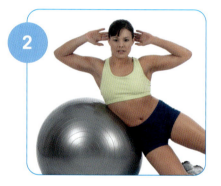

- Raise your upper body up and off the ball, bringing your outside elbow down to your side.

- Lower your body, returning to the starting position. Lie over the ball.

Intensity

Weight Loss	Toning
2 SETS	3 SETS
20 REPS	12 REPS
30-SECOND REST	30-SECOND REST
BETWEEN SETS	BETWEEN SETS

HINTS

Control the movement through your midsection. Move slowly, trying to avoid jerky movements. • Keep your upper body upright, and do not allow your shoulders to fall forward or your elbows to come together.

WORKOUT 1: Standing Hamstring Stretch

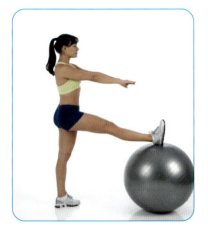

- Stand with one heel on the ball in front of you.

- Stretch your arms out in front of you, and gently bend forward at the waist, bringing your hands toward your foot.

Intensity

HOLD FOR 10 SECONDS
REPEAT 3 TIMES WITH EACH LEG

WORKOUT 1: Lying Quadriceps Stretch

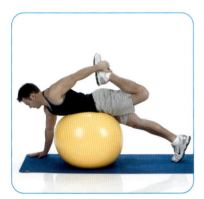

- Lie facedown over the ball, positioning it in your midsection. Start with both hands and feet on the floor.

- Raise one leg, bending at the knee, and hold the ankle with your hand.

- Pull your foot toward your buttocks.

Intensity

HOLD FOR 10 SECONDS
REPEAT 3 TIMES WITH EACH LEG

WORKOUT 1: Glute Stretch

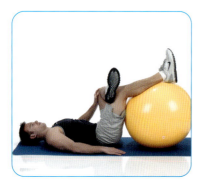

- Lie with your back on the mat. Place one leg on the ball with your knee bent.

- Place the other ankle across that knee. Gently push the outside knee away from you.

Intensity

HOLD FOR 10 SECONDS
REPEAT 3 TIMES WITH EACH LEG

WORKOUT 1: Supine Chest Stretch

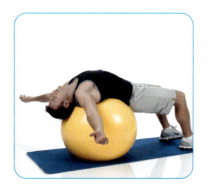

- Lie with your back on the ball and your arms stretched overhead.

- Roll back so the ball rests in your mid-back with your head, shoulders, and arms hanging over it. Lower your hands toward the floor.

Intensity

HOLD FOR 10 SECONDS
REPEAT 3 TIMES

WORKOUT 1: Spine Flexion Stretch

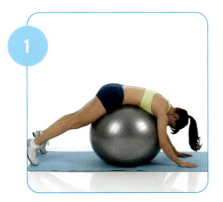

1

- Lie face down with the ball centered under your midsection.

- Place your hands and feet on the floor, and let your head and shoulders fall forward over the ball.

- Allow your spine to flex as you stretch over the ball.

Intensity

HOLD FOR 10 SECONDS
REPEAT 3 TIMES

WORKOUT 2: Squat to Ball

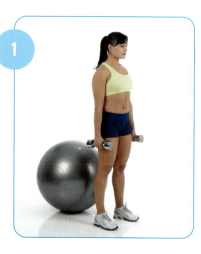

1

- Start with the ball behind you on the floor.

- Stand upright with a dumbbell in each hand with your feet facing forward about hip-width apart.

2

- Lower your body until you touch the ball.

- Keep your back in a neutral position.

- Push through your feet to return to the starting position.

Intensity

Weight Loss	Toning
2 SETS	3 SETS
20 REPS	12 REPS
30-SECOND REST	30-SECOND REST
BETWEEN SETS	BETWEEN SETS

HINTS

The position of your back is very important in squatting exercises. Always maintain a neutral spine position.
• Do not round your lower back or overarch it. • Keep your head up, looking forward with your shoulders pulled back. • You can position the ball against a wall so it will not move around as you move down and up.

WORKOUT 2: Kneeling Push-Up

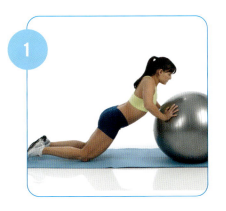

• Kneel on the mat with your hands on the ball, shoulder-width apart, with elbows bent and your chest nearly touching the ball.

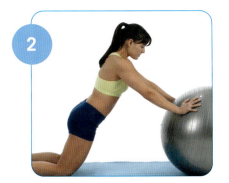

• Push up and away from the ball until your arms are fully extended. Keep your spine straight.

• Lower your body until your chest is almost touching the ball.

Intensity

Weight Loss	Toning
2 SETS	3 SETS
20 REPS	12 REPS
30-SECOND REST	30-SECOND REST
BETWEEN SETS	BETWEEN SETS

HINTS

Start with your feet on the floor to help with stability. • To increase difficulty, raise your feet off the floor so you are balanced on your knees. • Make sure to keep your upper body straight. Do not let your midsection sag or arch.

WORKOUT 2: Wide Row

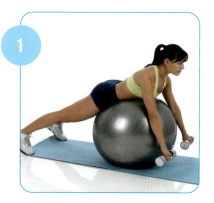

- Lie facedown over the ball, centering your mid-abdomen with your legs stretched out behind you.

- Hold a dumbbell in each hand with your arms extended over the front of the ball.

- Slightly bend your elbows, sticking them out to the sides.

- Your palms should face back to the ball.

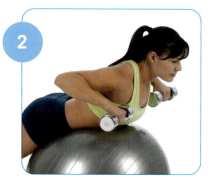

- Raise the dumbbells, drawing your shoulder blades together and bending your elbows outward.

- Lower the dumbbells back toward the floor, extending your elbows.

Intensity

Weight Loss	Toning
2 SETS	**3 SETS**
20 REPS	**12 REPS**
30-SECOND REST	**30-SECOND REST**
BETWEEN SETS	**BETWEEN SETS**

HINTS

Start with your feet about shoulder-width apart. • To increase the challenge to your stability, move your feet closer together. • Draw your elbows up and out to your sides, not in close. • Look down at the floor to keep your head in line with your spine. • Do not lift your head as you raise the dumbbells.

WORKOUT 2: Seated Lateral Raise

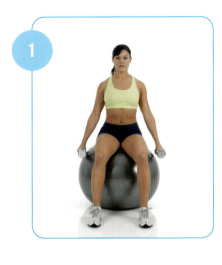

- Sit upright on the ball with your feet flat on the floor.

- Hold a dumbbell in each hand with your palms facing in and your arms extended by your sides.

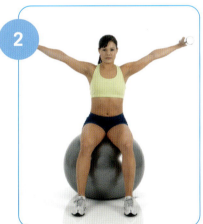

- Raise the dumbbells up and out from your sides. Raise them just above shoulder level, keeping your arms straight.

- Lower the dumbbells down to the starting position.

- Be sure to lower the dumbbells until your arms are fully extended by your sides.

Intensity

Weight Loss	Toning
2 SETS	3 SETS
20 REPS	12 REPS
30-SECOND REST	30-SECOND REST
BETWEEN SETS	BETWEEN SETS

HINTS

Keep your back upright by contracting your core muscles as you raise the dumbbells. • Move slowly and smoothly. • To avoid excess stress on shoulder joints, you can bend your elbows slightly. • Start with your feet shoulder-width apart. To increase the challenge, move your feet closer together.

WORKOUT 2: Seated Hammer Curl

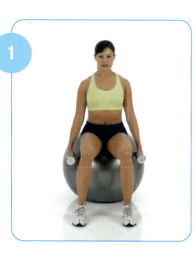

1

- Sit upright on the ball with your feet flat on the floor.

- Hold a dumbbell in each hand with your palms facing in and your arms extended by your sides.

2

- Raise the dumbbells in front to shoulder level, bending at the elbows.

- Lower the dumbbells by straightening your elbows and returning to the starting position.

- Be sure to lower the dumbbells until your arms are fully extended.

Intensity

Weight Loss	Toning
2 SETS	3 SETS
20 REPS	12 REPS
30-SECOND REST	30-SECOND REST
BETWEEN SETS	BETWEEN SETS

HINTS

Keep your back straight and aligned by contracting your core muscles. Do not round your lower back. •
Complete the full range of motion, from arms fully extended, to dumbbells at shoulder level, and back again.
• *Start with your feet shoulder-width apart. To increase the challenge, bring your feet closer together.*

WORKOUT 2: French Press

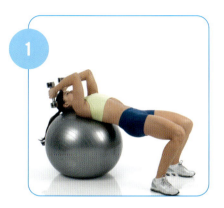

- Lie with your back over the ball in a reverse bridge position. Place the ball between your shoulder blades.

- Keep your hips level with your shoulders and your feet flat on the floor.

- Hold a dumbbell in each hand with your elbows flexed and the weights positioned at the sides of your head.

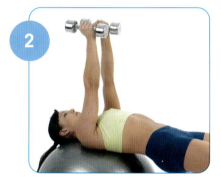

- Raise the dumbbells until your arms are straight and the weights are overhead.

- Lower the dumbbells by bending your elbows to return to the starting position.

- Make sure to go all the way down until the dumbbells are back at the sides of your head.

Intensity

Weight Loss	Toning
2 SETS	3 SETS
20 REPS	12 REPS
30-SECOND REST BETWEEN SETS	30-SECOND REST BETWEEN SETS

HINTS

Keep your hips in line with your shoulders. Do not let them sag or dip. This requires contracting your abdominals and lower back muscles. • Be careful not to hit yourself in the back of the head as you lift and lower the dumbbell. • Keep the shoulders steady. Do not allow your upper arm to move around; movement should only occur at the elbow joint.

WORKOUT 2: Crunch on Ball

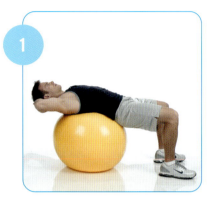

- Lie with your mid-back on the ball in a reverse bridge position.

- Keep your head and neck off the ball and your feet flat on the floor.

- Place your hands at the sides of your head.

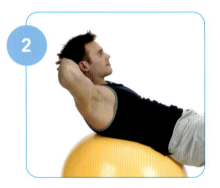

- Lift your head and shoulders up and away from the ball, contracting your abdominals.

- Roll your upper body back over the ball, returning to the starting position.

Intensity

Weight Loss	Toning
2 SETS	**3 SETS**
20 REPS	**12 REPS**
30-SECOND REST	**30-SECOND REST**
BETWEEN SETS	**BETWEEN SETS**

HINTS

Control the movement through your midsection and avoid jerky movements. • Do not use your hands to pull up your head and neck. • Lift only your head and shoulders. • Start with your feet shoulder-width apart. To increase the challenge to your stability, move your feet closer together.

WORKOUT 2: Lateral Bridge

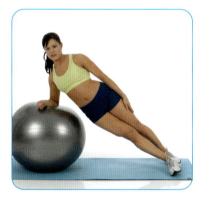

• Lie on one side with your forearm on the ball and your legs stretched out to one side.

• Position your other arm at your side.

• Lift your hips off the ball. Hold this position for 10 seconds, then lower your hips back down to the ball.

• Repeat according to your chosen intensity, then switch sides.

Intensity

Weight Loss	Toning
2 SETS	3 SETS
20 REPS	12 REPS
30-SECOND REST	30-SECOND REST
BETWEEN SETS	BETWEEN SETS

HINTS

Lie with your side on the ball. Raise your hips off the ball and hold this position. • Do not let your hips sag or dip. This will require you to contract the abdominal and core muscles. • Keep your upper body aligned with your hips. Do not allow your shoulders to fall forward. • Look straight ahead to maintain a neutral spine.

WORKOUT 2: Lying Hamstring Stretch

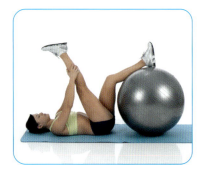

- Lie on your back on the mat. Place one leg on the ball with your knee bent.

- Keep the other leg straight, and clasp your hands behind your calf.

- Slowly pull the straight leg toward your head.

Intensity

HOLD FOR 10 SECONDS
REPEAT 3 TIMES WITH EACH LEG

WORKOUT 2: Standing Quadriceps Stretch

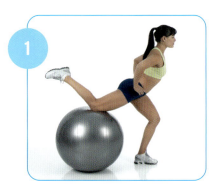

- Stand with one knee on the ball and the other foot in front.

- Gently lean forward, pushing your knee into the ball.

- For a more intense stretch, grasp the ankle of the leg on the ball and pull it toward your buttocks.

Intensity

HOLD FOR 10 SECONDS
REPEAT 3 TIMES WITH EACH LEG

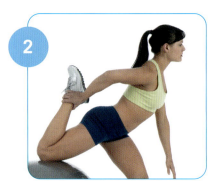

WORKOUT 2: Lying Hip Adductor Stretch

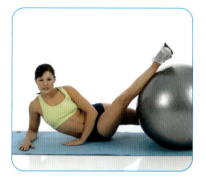

- Lie on your side with your lower leg on the ball and the other leg behind it.
- Push down on the ball with your leg, and raise your upper body off the mat.

Intensity

HOLD FOR 10 SECONDS
REPEAT 3 TIMES WITH EACH LEG

WORKOUT 2: Upper Back Stretch

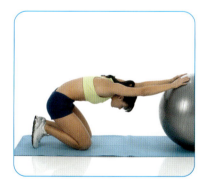

- Kneel on the floor with your hands on top of the ball at arm's length.
- Lower your head between your shoulders and arch your back.
- Sit back on your heels.

Intensity

HOLD FOR 10 SECONDS
REPEAT 3 TIMES

WORKOUT 2: Shoulder Stretch

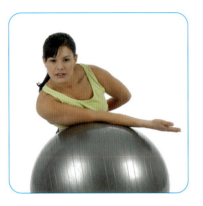

- Kneel on the floor with the ball in front of you with your upper arm resting on top of it.

- Lower your upper body toward the ball as you feel a stretch along the back of your shoulder.

Intensity

HOLD FOR 10 SECONDS
REPEAT 3 TIMES WITH EACH ARM

WORKOUT 3: Dead Lift to Ball Overhead

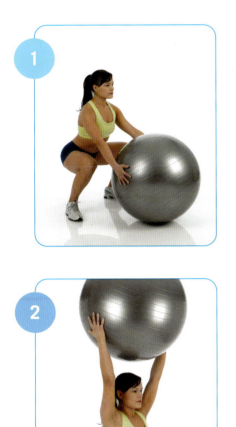

1
- Start in a squat position with your feet flat on the floor, head up, and your back in a neutral position.
- Hold the ball on the floor in front of you.

2
- Stand up and lift the ball overhead with your arms fully extended.
- Lower yourself back down so the ball is again on the floor in front of you.

Intensity

Weight Loss	Toning
2 SETS	3 SETS
20 REPS	12 REPS
30-SECOND REST	30-SECOND REST
BETWEEN SETS	BETWEEN SETS

HINTS

Your back position is very important in squatting exercises. Always maintain a neutral position. • Do not round your lower back or overarch it. • Keep your head up, looking straight ahead with your shoulders pulled back throughout the exercise.

WORKOUT 3: Incline Chest Press

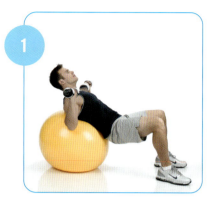

- Lie back on the ball in a reverse bridge position. The ball should be centered between your shoulder blades.

- Drop your hips so your back rests on the ball and your body is at a 45-degree angle, with your feet flat on the floor.

- Hold a dumbbell in each hand at shoulder level.

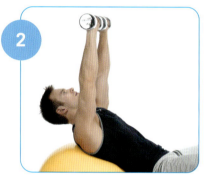

- Lift the dumbbells until your arms are straight, and the dumbbells are directly over your upper chest.

- Lower the dumbbells by bending your elbows to return to the starting position.

- Be sure to lower the dumbbells back to shoulder level.

Intensity

Weight Loss	Toning
2 SETS	3 SETS
20 REPS	12 REPS
30-SECOND REST	30-SECOND REST
BETWEEN SETS	BETWEEN SETS

HINTS

Although your hips and back are on the ball, keep your abdominal muscles contracted to stabilize you. • Keep the dumbbells directly over your chest. Do not let them move outward or inward. • Start with your feet about shoulder-width apart. To challenge your stability, bring your feet closer together.

WORKOUT 3: Lateral Rollout

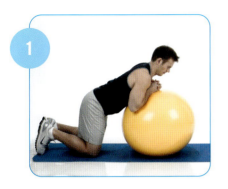

• Kneel on the mat with your forearms on the ball, your elbows bent, and your chest nearly touching the ball.

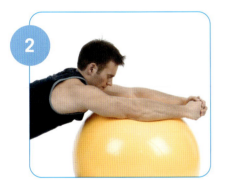

• Push the ball forward, extending your arms and keeping your upper body rigid.

• Pull the ball back, drawing your elbows in until you reach the starting position.

Intensity

Weight Loss	Toning
2 SETS	3 SETS
20 REPS	12 REPS
30-SECOND REST	30-SECOND REST
BETWEEN SETS	BETWEEN SETS

HINTS

Maintain a neutral spine by looking down and not moving your head. • Control the movement through your midsection, and avoid jerky movements. This requires you to keep your abdominal and core muscles contracted throughout the exercise.

WORKOUT 3: Seated Upright Row

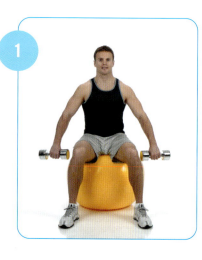

1

- Sit upright on the ball with your feet flat on the floor.

- Hold a dumbbell in each hand with your palms facing backward and your arms by your sides.

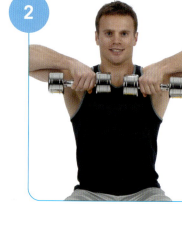

2

- Raise the dumbbells to a position under your chin, moving your elbows above your shoulders.

- Lower the dumbbells to the starting position, extended by your sides.

Intensity

Weight Loss	Toning
2 SETS	3 SETS
20 REPS	12 REPS
30-SECOND REST	30-SECOND REST
BETWEEN SETS	BETWEEN SETS

HINTS

When lifting the dumbbells, make sure to raise your elbows higher than your shoulders. • Do not turn your wrists; keep the dumbbells level throughout the exercise. Bring them close together at the top of the extension without banging them together.

WORKOUT 3: Seated Twisting Curl

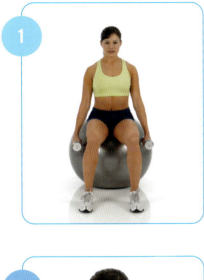

1

- Sit upright on the ball with your feet flat on the floor.

- Hold a dumbbell in each hand with your palms facing in and your arms extended by your sides.

2

- Raise the dumbbells in front to shoulder level, bending your elbows and twisting at the wrist so your palms face back.

- Lower the dumbbells, straightening your elbows, and returning to the starting position.

- Finish the exercise so your arms are again fully extended.

Intensity

Weight Loss	Toning
2 SETS	3 SETS
20 REPS	12 REPS
30-SECOND REST	30-SECOND REST
BETWEEN SETS	BETWEEN SETS

HINTS

Keep your back upright by contracting your core muscles. Do not round your lower back. • *Complete the full range of motion, from arms fully extended, to dumbbells at shoulder level, and back again.* • *Start with your feet about shoulder-width apart. To challenge your stability, bring your feet closer together.*

WORKOUT 3: Dips with Hands on Ball

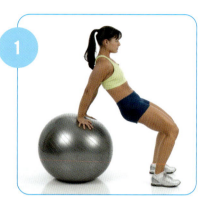

- With the ball behind you, place your hands on top of it with your arms straight. Keep your feet flat on the floor in front and bend your knees slightly.

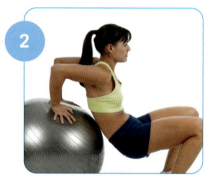

- Lower your body toward the floor by bending your elbows and dropping until your lower back touches the ball.

- Push up against the ball to the starting position with your arms fully extended.

- Keep your feet flat on the floor throughout the entire movement.

Intensity

Weight Loss	Toning
2 SETS	3 SETS
20 REPS	12 REPS
30-SECOND REST	30-SECOND REST
BETWEEN SETS	BETWEEN SETS

HINTS

Position the ball against a wall to prevent it from moving around. • *Do not sit on the ball in the lower position; barely touch the ball with your lower back.* • *To increase difficulty, straighten your legs, and place your heels on the floor.* • *Keep your head up and look straight ahead.*

WORKOUT 3: Weighted Crunch

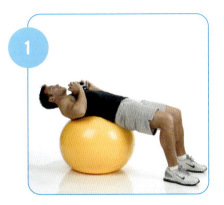

- Lie across the ball with your back in a reverse bridge position, centering the ball in your mid-back.

- Keep your head and neck off the ball.

- Hold a dumbbell in both hands under your chin and close to your chest.

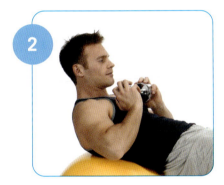

- Lift your head and shoulders up and away from the ball, contracting your abdominals.

- Roll your upper body back over the ball, returning to the starting position. Hold the dumbbell in the same position throughout the exercise.

Intensity

Weight Loss	Toning
2 SETS	3 SETS
20 REPS	12 REPS
30-SECOND REST	30-SECOND REST
BETWEEN SETS	BETWEEN SETS

HINTS

Control the movement through your midsection, and avoid jerky movements. • Keep the weight close to your chest, holding it in your hands. • Lift only your head and shoulders, not your whole back. • Start with your feet shoulder-width apart. To make it more challenging, bring your feet closer together.

WORKOUT 3: Lower Body Twist

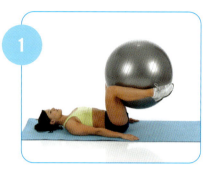

- Lie with your back on the mat. Place the ball between your feet, and raise it off the floor with your knees bent.

- Place your hands at your sides on the mat.

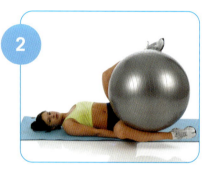

- Rotate your lower body, shifting your knee to one side until it touches the floor, keeping the ball between your feet.

- Rotate 180 degrees to the other side, touching the floor with the other knee.

Intensity

Weight Loss	Toning
2 SETS	3 SETS
20 REPS	12 REPS
30-SECOND REST	30-SECOND REST
BETWEEN SETS	BETWEEN SETS

HINTS

Keep your shoulders and upper back on the mat throughout the exercise. • Twist through your midsection, using your abdominal muscles to move you.

WORKOUT 3: Standing Hamstring Stretch

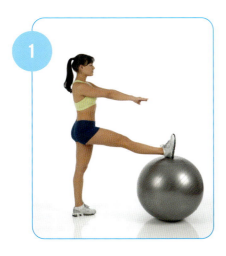

• Stand with one heel on the ball in front of you.

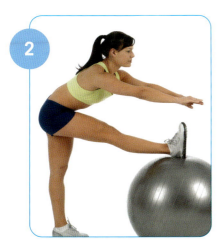

• Stretch your arms out in front of you and gently lean forward at the waist, moving your hands toward your foot.

Intensity

HOLD FOR 10 SECONDS
REPEAT 3 TIMES WITH EACH LEG

WORKOUT 3: Hip Flexor Stretch

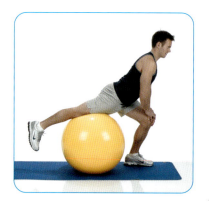

- Stand over the ball with one leg in front and the other behind you.

- Shift your body weight forward, stretching the back hip joint.

Intensity

HOLD FOR 10 SECONDS
REPEAT 3 TIMES WITH EACH LEG

WORKOUT 3: Lying Hip Abductor Stretch

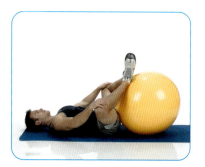

- Lie with your back on the mat and the ball in front of you.

- Place your ankles on the ball, keeping your heels together.

- Gently push your knees away from your body and toward the ball.

Intensity

HOLD FOR 10 SECONDS
REPEAT 3 TIMES

WORKOUT 3: One-Sided Chest Stretch

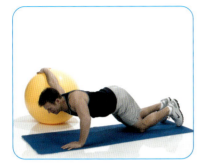

- Kneel on all fours with the ball to one side of you.

- Place your hand on top of the ball with your arm extended.

- Lower your body into a stretch across your upper chest.

Intensity

HOLD FOR 10 SECONDS

REPEAT 3 TIMES WITH EACH ARM

WORKOUT 3: Lateral Stretch

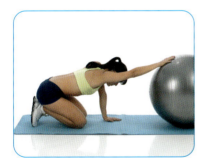

- Kneel on the floor with one hand on top of the ball positioned at arm's length.

- Keep your head down and look at the floor. Sit back on your heels.

- Lower your shoulder toward the floor until you feel the stretch along the side of your back.

Intensity

HOLD FOR 10 SECONDS

REPEAT 3 TIMES WITH EACH ARM

WORKOUT 4: Lateral Lunge with Ball Overhead

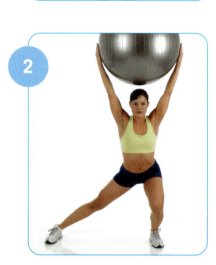

1 • Stand upright with your feet about hip-width apart, and hold the ball at waist height.

2 • Step laterally to one side, and lower your body to a half-squat position. Lift the ball overhead with your arms fully extended.

• Push off the outside foot to return to your starting position, and lower the ball back to waist height.

• Repeat the exercise with the other leg.

Intensity

Weight Loss	Toning
2 SETS	**3 SETS**
20 REPS	**12 REPS**
30-SECOND REST	**30-SECOND REST**
BETWEEN SETS	**BETWEEN SETS**

HINTS

The back position is very important in squatting exercises. Always maintain a neutral position. Do not round your lower back or overarch it. • Keep your head up, looking straight ahead with your shoulders back. • Place your body's weight over your active foot and push off this leg to regain an upright standing position. • Keep the other leg straight throughout the exercise.

WORKOUT 4: Reciprocal Chest Press

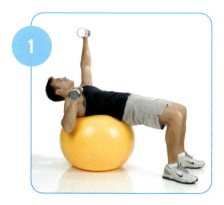

- Lie with your back on the ball in a reverse bridge position. Center the ball between your shoulder blades.

- Keep your hips level with your shoulders and your feet flat on the floor.

- Hold a dumbbell in each hand, with one at shoulder level, and the other with a fully extended arm.

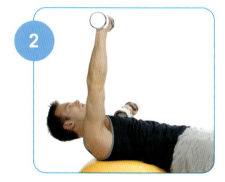

- Lift one dumbbell to a straight-arm position directly over your upper chest, as you lower the other to shoulder level in a reciprocal motion.

- Lower the dumbbell by bending at the elbow and returning it to shoulder level as you lift the other dumbbell to the straight-arm position.

Intensity

Weight Loss	Toning
2 SETS	3 SETS
20 REPS	12 REPS
30-SECOND REST	30-SECOND REST
BETWEEN SETS	BETWEEN SETS

HINTS

Keep your hips in line with your shoulders. Do not let them sag or dip. This requires you to contract your abdominal and core muscles. • Move both dumbbells at the same time in a smooth balanced motion. • Keep the dumbbells directly over your chest. Do not let them move outward or inward. • Start with your feet shoulder-width apart. To make the exercise more challenging, bring your feet closer together.

WORKOUT 4: Single-Arm Close Row

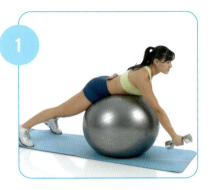

1

- Lie face down over the ball with it under your mid-abdomen and your legs stretched out behind you.

- Hold a dumbbell in one hand with your arm extended in front of the ball and your elbow slightly bent, with your palm facing in.

- Place your other hand behind your back.

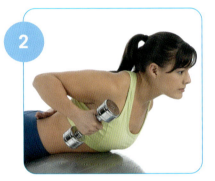

2

- Lift the dumbbell by drawing your shoulder blade to the center of your back and bending your elbow.

- Lower the dumbbell back to the starting position, extending it at the elbow.

Intensity

Weight Loss	Toning
2 SETS	**3 SETS**
20 REPS	**12 REPS**
30-SECOND REST	**30-SECOND REST**
BETWEEN SETS	**BETWEEN SETS**

HINTS

Start with your feet shoulder-width apart. To make it more challenging, bring your feet closer together. • Draw your elbow up along your side, not outward. • Look down at the floor to keep your head aligned with your spine. Do not lift your head as you raise the dumbbell. • Do desired sets with both arms.

WORKOUT 4: Seated Leg Extension

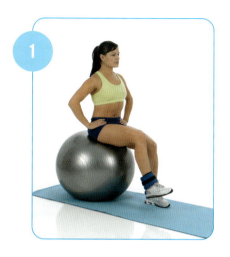

- Sit upright on the ball with weights on each ankle and your feet flat on the floor.

- Place your hands on your hips.

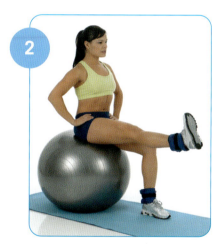

- Lift one foot off the floor and extend your leg straight out in front of you.

- Lower your leg, bending at the knee and return to the starting position with both feet on the floor.

- Repeat the exercise with the other leg.

Intensity

Weight Loss	Toning
2 SETS	3 SETS
20 REPS	12 REPS
30-SECOND REST	30-SECOND REST
BETWEEN SETS	BETWEEN SETS

HINTS

Keep your back upright by contracting your core muscles as you raise your leg. Do not round your lower back.
• Keep one foot on the floor throughout the movement to maintain stability. • Place your hands on your hips and look straight ahead to keep your head and upper body level.

WORKOUT 4: Seated Front Raise

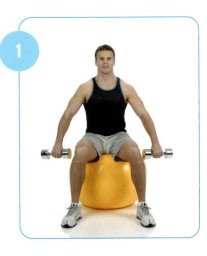

1

- Sit upright on the ball with your feet flat on the floor.

- Hold a dumbbell in each hand with your palms facing down and your arms extended by your sides.

2

- Lift the dumbbells to just above shoulder level, keeping your arms straight.

- Lower the dumbbells down to your sides, returning to the starting position. Be sure to lower your arms until they are fully extended.

Intensity

Weight Loss	Toning
2 SETS	**3 SETS**
20 REPS	**12 REPS**
30-SECOND REST	**30-SECOND REST**
BETWEEN SETS	**BETWEEN SETS**

HINTS

Keep your back upright by contracting your core muscles as you raise the dumbbells. • *Avoid jerky movements.* • *Bend your elbows slightly to avoid excess stress on shoulder joints.* • *Start with your feet shoulder-width apart. To make it more challenging, bring your feet closer together.*

WORKOUT 4: Single-Arm Hammer Curl

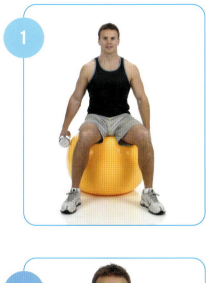

- Sit upright on the ball with your feet flat on the floor.

- Hold a dumbbell in one hand, with your palm facing in, and your arms extended along your sides.

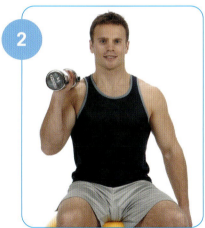

- Raise the dumbbell in front to shoulder level by bending your elbow.

- Lower the dumbbell by straightening your elbow to return to the starting position.

- Keep the other arm by your side throughout the movement.

- Repeat according to your chosen intensity, then switch sides.

Intensity

Weight Loss	Toning
2 SETS	3 SETS
20 REPS	12 REPS
30-SECOND REST	30-SECOND REST
BETWEEN SETS	BETWEEN SETS

HINTS

Keep your back upright by contracting your core muscles. Do not round your lower back. • Complete the full range of motion, from arm fully extended, to dumbbell at shoulder level, and back again. • Start with your feet shoulder-width apart. To make it more challenging, bring your feet closer together.

WORKOUT 4: Double-Arm Triceps Extension

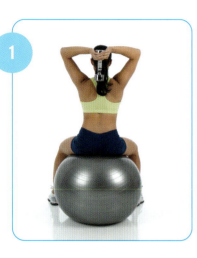

1

- Sit upright on the ball with your feet flat on the floor.
- Hold the end of the dumbbell behind your head with both hands and your elbows bent.

2

- Lift the dumbbell by extending your elbows and straightening your arms directly overhead.
- Lower the dumbbell by bending at the elbows, returning to the starting position with the dumbbells behind your head.

Intensity

Weight Loss	Toning
2 SETS	3 SETS
20 REPS	12 REPS
30-SECOND REST	30-SECOND REST
BETWEEN SETS	BETWEEN SETS

HINTS

Keep your back upright by contracting your core muscles. Do not round your lower back. • Be careful not to hit the back of your head as you lift and lower the dumbbell. • Complete the full range of motion, from behind the head, to the arm fully extended overhead, and back again. • Keep your upper arms and shoulders steady. Movement should occur only at the elbows.

WORKOUT 4: Crunch with Rotation

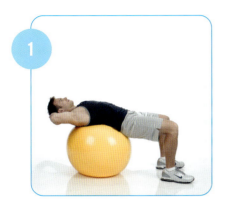

- Lie across the ball in a reverse bridge position, centering the ball in your mid-back.

- Keep your head and neck off the ball and your feet flat on the floor.

- Place your hands at the sides of your head.

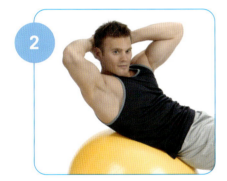

- Lift your head and shoulders up and away from the ball, and rotate them to one side by contracting your abdominals and twisting through your midsection.

- Twist back to the center and roll your upper body back over the ball, returning to the starting position.

Intensity

Weight Loss	Toning
2 SETS	3 SETS
20 REPS	12 REPS
30-SECOND REST	30-SECOND REST
BETWEEN SETS	BETWEEN SETS

HINTS

Control the movement through your midsection, and avoid jerky movements. • Do not use your hands to pull your head and neck up. • Lift only your head and shoulders, not your whole back. • Start with your feet shoulder-width apart. To make it more challenging, bring your feet closer together.

WORKOUT 4: Bridge with Feet on Ball

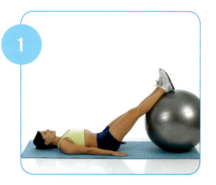

- Lie with your back on the mat and your heels on top of the ball.

- Place your hands by your sides on the mat.

- Lift your hips off the mat by contracting your core and abdominal muscles, and hold this position for 10 seconds.

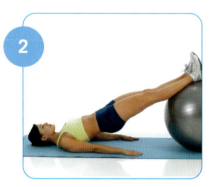

- After holding for 10 seconds, lower your body back to the mat, returning to the starting position.

- Repeat this movement, holding at the top for each repetition.

Intensity

Weight Loss	Toning
2 SETS	3 SETS
20 REPS	12 REPS
30-SECOND REST	30-SECOND REST
BETWEEN SETS	BETWEEN SETS

HINTS

Keep your core and abdominal muscles contracted and maintain a neutral spine throughout the movement.
• Use your hands to help stabilize yourself by pushing them into floor when raising your hips. • Only your head, upper back, and shoulders should touch the mat at the top position.

WORKOUT 4: Oblique Crunch

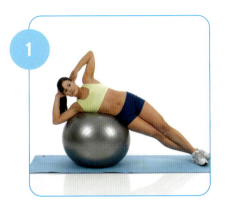

- Lie with your side on the ball with both legs extended and your feet on the mat.

- Place your hands at the sides of your head.

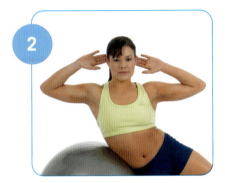

- Raise your upper body up and off the ball, bringing your outside elbow down to your side.

- Lower your body, returning to the starting position lying over the ball.

Intensity

Weight Loss	Toning
2 SETS	3 SETS
20 REPS	12 REPS
30-SECOND REST	30-SECOND REST
BETWEEN SETS	BETWEEN SETS

HINTS

Control the movement through your midsection and avoid jerky movements. • Keep your upper body upright. Do not allow your shoulders to fall forward or your elbows to come together.

WORKOUT 4: Lying Hamstring Stretch

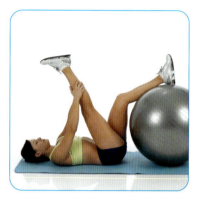

- Lie with your back on the mat. Place one leg on the ball with your knee bent.

- Keep the other leg straight, and clasp your hands behind your calf.

- Slowly pull the straight leg toward your head.

Intensity

HOLD FOR 10 SECONDS
REPEAT 3 TIMES WITH EACH LEG

WORKOUT 4: Glute Stretch

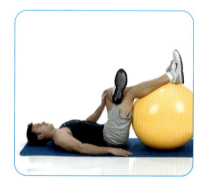

- Lie with your back on the mat. Place one foot on the ball with your knee bent.

- Place the other foot on that knee. Gently push the outside knee away from you.

Intensity

HOLD FOR 10 SECONDS
REPEAT 3 TIMES WITH EACH LEG

WORKOUT 4: Standing Hip Abductor Stretch

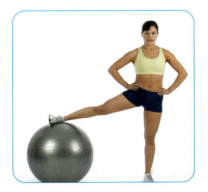

- Stand with the inside ankle of one leg on the ball.
- Slowly lower your body, stretching the inside of the leg on the ball.

Intensity

HOLD FOR 10 SECONDS
REPEAT 3 TIMES WITH EACH LEG

WORKOUT 4: Lateral Spine Flexion Stretch

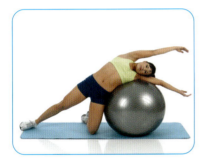

- Kneel beside the ball with your arms extended overhead.
- Lean over the ball as you extend your far leg straight.

Intensity

HOLD FOR 10 SECONDS
REPEAT 3 TIMES ON EACH SIDE

WORKOUT 4: Triceps Stretch

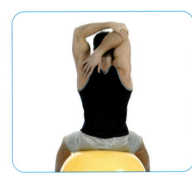

- Sit upright on the ball with one arm, bent at the elbow, behind your head.
- Place the other hand on that elbow, and slowly pull it across to the middle of your back.

Intensity

HOLD FOR 10 SECONDS
REPEAT 3 TIMES WITH EACH ARM

WORKOUT 5: Squat to Ball

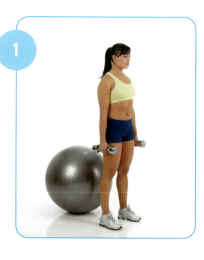

1

- Start with the ball on the floor behind you.

- Stand upright with a dumbbell in each hand, and stand facing forward with your feet hip-width apart.

2

- Lower your body to the ball until you just touch it.

- Keep your back in a neutral position.

- Push through your feet to return to the starting position.

Intensity

Weight Loss	Toning
2 SETS	3 SETS
20 REPS	12 REPS
30-SECOND REST	30-SECOND REST
BETWEEN SETS	BETWEEN SETS

HINTS

Back position is very important in squatting exercises. Always maintain it in a neutral position. Do not round your lower back or overarch it. • Keep your head up, looking straight ahead with your shoulders back. • You can position the ball against the wall on the floor so it will not move.

WORKOUT 5: Reciprocal Incline Chest Press

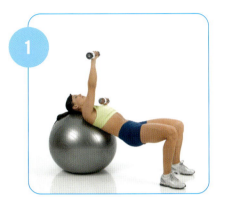

- Lie with your back on the ball in a reverse bridge position with the ball squarely between your shoulder blades.

- Drop your hips so your back rests on the ball, and your body is at a 45-degree angle with your feet flat on the floor.

- Hold a dumbbell in each hand: one at shoulder level and the other with a fully extended arm.

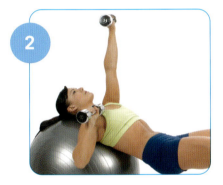

- Press one dumbbell up to a straight-arm position directly over your upper chest as you lower the other to shoulder level in a reciprocal motion.

- Lower the dumbbell by bending at your elbow. Return it to shoulder level, as you press the other dumbbell up to the straight-arm position.

Intensity

Weight Loss	Toning
2 SETS	3 SETS
20 REPS	12 REPS
30-SECOND REST	30-SECOND REST
BETWEEN SETS	BETWEEN SETS

HINTS

Although your hips and back are on the ball, keep your abdominal muscles contracted for stability. • Move both dumbbells at the same time in a smooth reciprocal action. • Keep the dumbbells directly over your chest.• Start with your feet shoulder-width apart. To challenge your stability further, bring your feet closer together.

WORKOUT 5: Bent-Over Row

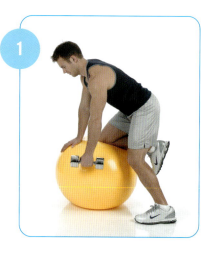

- Choose either your right or left side, and place that knee and hand on the ball.

- Hold a dumbbell in the other hand, with your arm fully extended by your side.

- Place the other foot flat on the floor a little behind and to the side of the ball.

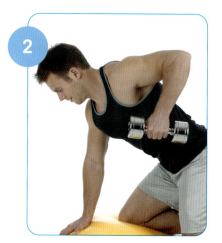

- Raise the dumbbell to your chest, bending at the elbow.

- Lower the dumbbell back to the starting position, keeping your back neutral throughout the entire movement.

Intensity

Weight Loss	Toning
2 SETS	3 SETS
20 REPS	12 REPS
30-SECOND REST	30-SECOND REST
BETWEEN SETS	BETWEEN SETS

HINTS

Look toward the floor to maintain a neutral spine. • Do not lift your head as you lift the dumbbell. • Raise the dumbbell so your elbow travels above your shoulder height.

WORKOUT 5: Prone Hamstring Curls

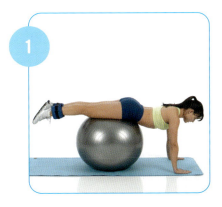

- With weights on each ankle, lie facedown with the ball under your upper legs.

- Extend your arms and place your hands on the mat directly under your shoulders.

- Your body should be in a straight line from head to feet.

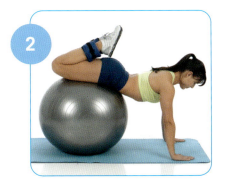

- Bending at the knees, bring both feet to your buttocks.

- Extend your legs, lowering your feet back to the starting position.

Intensity

Weight Loss	Toning
2 SETS	3 SETS
20 REPS	12 REPS
30-SECOND REST	30-SECOND REST
BETWEEN SETS	BETWEEN SETS

HINTS

To maintain a neutral spine, look at the floor and do not raise your head during the exercise. • Keep your arms fully extended throughout the movement. • Move your feet in to touch your buttocks and out to a straight-leg position.

WORKOUT 5: Reciprocal Overhead Press

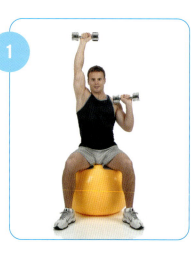

- Sit upright on the ball with your feet flat on the floor.

- Hold a dumbbell in each hand: one at shoulder level and the other overhead with your arm fully extended.

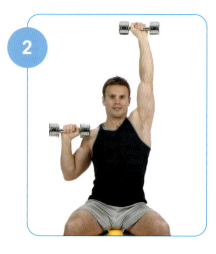

- Lift one dumbbell as you lower the other in a reciprocal motion.

- Lower the dumbbell by bending your elbow and dropping it to shoulder level. Simultaneously, press the other dumbbell up to the straight-arm position.

Intensity

Weight Loss	Toning
2 SETS	3 SETS
20 REPS	12 REPS
30-SECOND REST	30-SECOND REST
BETWEEN SETS	BETWEEN SETS

HINTS

Keep your back upright by contracting your core muscles as you push the dumbbells overhead. Do not round your lower back. • Complete the full range of motion: from shoulder level, to arms fully extended overhead, and back again. • Both dumbbells should be moving at the same time in a smooth, balanced motion. • Start with your feet shoulder-width apart. To make it more challenging, bring your feet closer together.

WORKOUT 5: Preacher Curl

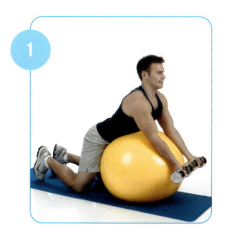

- Kneel on the mat with your chest and elbows on the ball, and your arms fully extended over the ball. Hold a dumbbell in each hand with palms facing up.

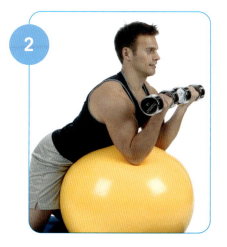

- Raise the dumbbells to shoulder level, bending at the elbows.

- Lower the dumbbells by straightening your elbows, returning to the starting position with your arms fully extended over the ball.

Intensity

Weight Loss	Toning
2 SETS	**3 SETS**
20 REPS	**12 REPS**
30-SECOND REST	**30-SECOND REST**
BETWEEN SETS	**BETWEEN SETS**

HINTS

Keep your shoulders and upper arms steady by pressing your elbows into the ball. • *Be careful not to round your upper back as you curl up.* • *Maintain a neutral spine throughout the movement.*

WORKOUT 5: French Press

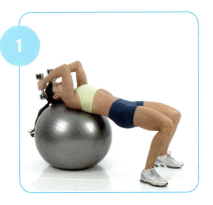

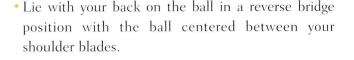

- Lie with your back on the ball in a reverse bridge position with the ball centered between your shoulder blades.

- Keep your hips level with your shoulders and your feet flat on the floor.

- Hold a dumbbell in each hand with your elbows bent and the weights positioned at the sides of your head.

- Raise the dumbbells until your arms are straight and the weights are overhead.

- Lower the dumbbells, bending at the elbows to return to the starting position, back at the sides of your head.

Intensity

Weight Loss	Toning
2 SETS	3 SETS
20 REPS	12 REPS
30-SECOND REST	30-SECOND REST
BETWEEN SETS	BETWEEN SETS

HINTS

Keep your hips in line with your shoulders. Do not let them sag or dip. This requires you to contract your abdominal and core muscles. • *Be careful not to hit the back of your head with the dumbbells as you lift and lower them.* • *Do not allow your upper arm to move around. Keep your shoulders steady; movement should occur only at the elbows.*

WORKOUT 5: Reverse Crunch

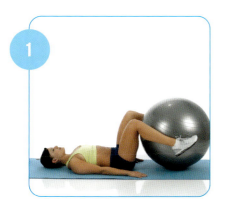

- Lie back on the mat. Position the ball on the mat between your feet with your knees bent.

- Place your hands at your sides.

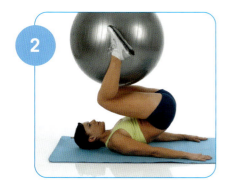

- Raise your hips and lower back off the mat, bringing your knees to your chest, and lifting the ball up.

- Return to the starting position with the ball on the mat.

Intensity

Weight Loss	Toning
2 SETS	3 SETS
20 REPS	12 REPS
30-SECOND REST	30-SECOND REST
BETWEEN SETS	BETWEEN SETS

HINTS

Keep your upper back and shoulders on the mat. • Do not move your legs. Keep your knees bent at the same angle throughout the exercise. • Complete the full range of motion, returning the ball to the mat every time.

WORKOUT 5: Single-Leg Reverse Bridge

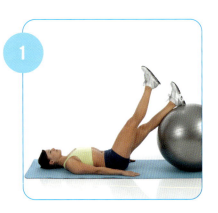

1

- Lie on your back on the mat with your heels on the ball and legs extended.

- Place your hands by your sides, and raise one foot off the ball.

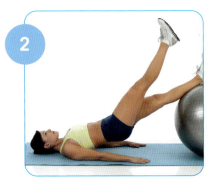

2

- Raise your hips off the mat, contracting your abdominals, and hold this position.

- Lower your hips back to the mat, returning to the starting position, keeping one leg off the ball.

Intensity

Weight Loss	Toning
2 SETS	**3 SETS**
20 REPS	**12 REPS**
30-SECOND REST	**30-SECOND REST**
BETWEEN SETS	**BETWEEN SETS**

HINTS

Keep your core and abdominal muscles contracted to maintain a neutral spine throughout the exercise. • Use your hands to help stabilize yourself by pushing them into the floor when raising your hips. • Only your head, upper back, and shoulders should touch the mat at the top position.

WORKOUT 5: Hip Raises

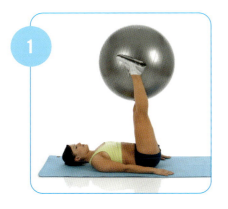

- Lie on your back on the mat with the ball between your feet and your legs straight up.

- Place your hands at your sides.

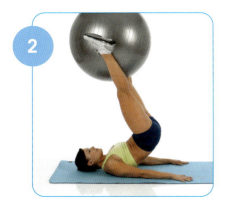

- Raise your hips and lower back off the mat, pushing the ball up.

- Return to the starting position with your hips and lower legs on the mat, and your legs straight up.

Intensity

Weight Loss	Toning
2 SETS	3 SETS
20 REPS	12 REPS
30-SECOND REST	30-SECOND REST
BETWEEN SETS	BETWEEN SETS

HINTS

Keep your upper back and shoulders on the mat. • Do not move your legs. Keep them straight throughout the movement. • Use your hands to help stabilize yourself by pushing them into the floor when raising your hips. • At the top position, only your head, shoulders, and upper back should touch the mat.

WORKOUT 5: Standing Hamstring Stretch

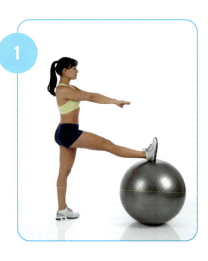

- Stand with one heel resting on the ball in front of you.

- Extend your arms out in front of you, and gently lean forward at the waist, stretching your hands toward your foot.

Intensity

HOLD FOR 10 SECONDS
REPEAT 3 TIMES WITH EACH LEG

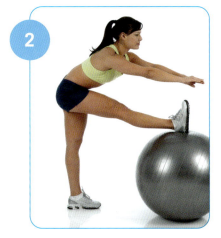

WORKOUT 5: **Standing Quadriceps Stretch**

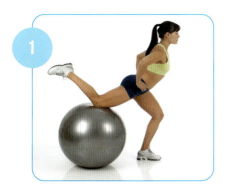

- Stand with one knee on the ball and the other foot in front of the ball.

- Gently lean forward, pushing your knee into the ball.

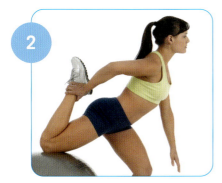

- For a more intense stretch, grasp the ankle of the leg on the ball and pull it toward your buttocks.

Intensity

HOLD FOR 10 SECONDS
REPEAT 3 TIMES WITH EACH LEG

WORKOUT 5: **Lying Hip Abductor Stretch**

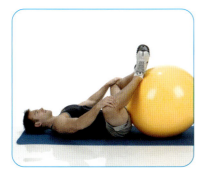

- Lie on your back on the mat with the ball in front of you.

- Place your ankles on the ball with your heels together, and gently push your knees away from your body.

Intensity

HOLD FOR 10 SECONDS
REPEAT 3 TIMES WITH EACH LEG

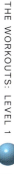

WORKOUT 5: Spinal Rotation Stretch

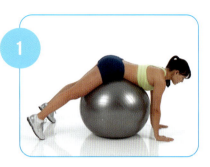

- Lie facedown over the ball, centering your midsection, and your feet and hands on the floor.

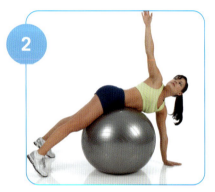

- Raise one arm and rotate at your waist until your arm is overhead and directly in line with the hand on the floor. Look up at the hand overhead.

Intensity

HOLD FOR 10 SECONDS
REPEAT 3 TIMES ON EACH SIDE

WORKOUT 5: Supine Chest Stretch

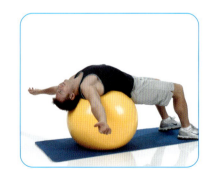

- Lie on your back over the ball and your arms stretched overhead.

- Roll back on the ball so it rests in your mid-back with your head, shoulders, and arms hanging down over the ball. Lower your hands towards the floor.

Intensity

HOLD FOR 10 SECONDS
REPEAT 3 TIMES

WORKOUT 1: Step-Up with Ball Overhead

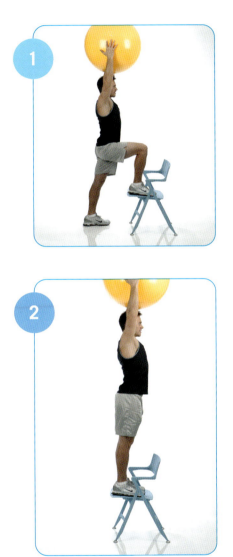

- Start with your arms fully extended overhead, holding the ball in your hands.

- Place one foot on a chair, keeping the other foot flat on the floor.

- Lean forward, shifting your body weight onto the foot on the chair.

- Push down on the foot on the chair, and using your core muscles, step up.

- Keep the ball overhead with your arms fully extended.

Intensity

Weight Loss	Toning
2 SETS	3 SETS
15 REPS	10 REPS
30-SECOND REST	30-SECOND REST
BETWEEN SETS	BETWEEN SETS

HINTS

Keep your head up and look straight ahead to maintain a neutral spine. • Put your weight on the foot on the chair not on the back foot. • Try not to push off using the back foot. Use the top leg to do the work.

WORKOUT 1: Push-Up with Feet on Ball

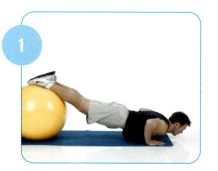

• Place your hands on the mat directly under your shoulders and position your feet on the ball.

• Your chest should nearly touch the mat with your body straight.

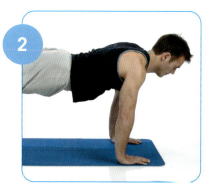

• Push up and away from the mat, extending your arms fully.

• Lower your body down to the mat until your chest is once again nearly touching it.

Intensity

Weight Loss	Toning
2 SETS	3 SETS
15 REPS	10 REPS
30-SECOND REST	30-SECOND REST
BETWEEN SETS	BETWEEN SETS

HINTS

Start by lying on your stomach on the ball and walking your hands out while rolling the ball down your legs to your feet. Go all the way down until your chest is nearly touching the mat, and then push back up, extending your arms fully. • Look down at the floor to maintain a neutral spine. Do not move your head.

WORKOUT 1: Lateral Rollout

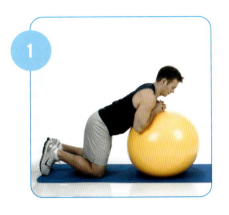

- Kneel on the mat with your forearms on the ball, elbows bent, and your chest nearly touching the ball.

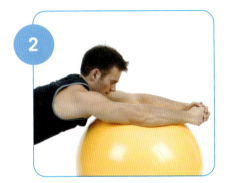

- Push the ball forward, extending your arms and keeping your upper body straight.

- Pull the ball back, drawing your elbows in until you reach your starting position.

Intensity

Weight Loss	Toning
2 SETS	3 SETS
15 REPS	10 REPS
30-SECOND REST	30-SECOND REST
BETWEEN SETS	BETWEEN SETS

HINTS

Maintain a neutral spine by looking down and not moving your head. • Control the movement through your midsection. Moving smoothly requires you to keep your abdominal and core muscles contracted.

WORKOUT 1: Hip Abduction

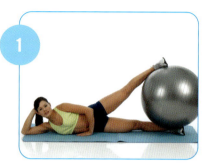

- Lie on your side on the mat with your legs extended and the ball between your feet.

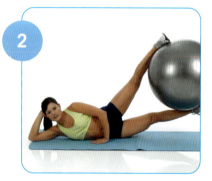

- Lift your legs, gripping the ball, up off the mat.

- Lower your legs and the ball, returning to your starting position.

- Repeat exercise on the other side.

Intensity

Weight Loss	Toning
2 SETS	3 SETS
15 REPS	10 REPS
30-SECOND REST	30-SECOND REST
BETWEEN SETS	BETWEEN SETS

HINTS

Use your arms to support yourself as you lift your legs. • Try to lift the ball as high as possible. • Keep your upper body and shoulders in line with your hips, and do not fall forward.

WORKOUT 1: **Single-Arm Overhead Press**

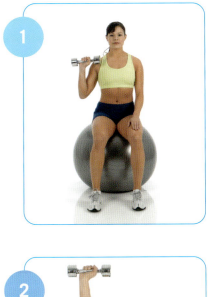

- Sit upright on the ball with your feet flat on the floor.

- Hold a dumbbell in one hand at shoulder level. Keep the other hand and arm at your side.

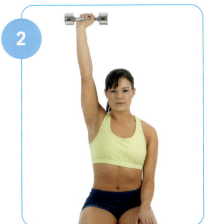

- Extending your arm, raise the dumbbell overhead.

- Bend your elbow to lower the dumbbell, and return to your starting position.

- Be sure to lower the dumbbell to shoulder level.

- Repeat on your other side.

Intensity

Weight Loss	*Toning*
2 SETS	**3 SETS**
15 REPS	**10 REPS**
30-SECOND REST	**30-SECOND REST**
BETWEEN SETS	**BETWEEN SETS**

HINTS

Keep your back upright by contracting your core muscles as you lift the dumbbell overhead. Do not round your lower back. • Complete the full range of motion from shoulder level, to arm fully extended overhead, and back again. • Start with your feet shoulder-width apart. To make it more challenging, bring your feet closer together.

WORKOUT 1: Single-Arm Straight Curl

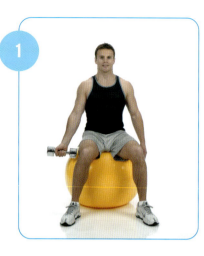

- Sit upright on the ball with your feet flat on the floor.

- Hold a dumbbell in one hand with your palm facing forward and your arms extended at your sides.

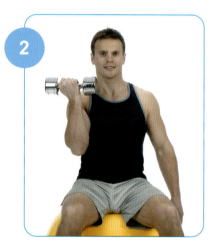

- Raise the dumbbell to shoulder level, by bending your elbow.

- Lower the dumbbell to the starting position at your side.

- Keep the other arm at your side throughout the movement.

Intensity

Weight Loss	Toning
2 SETS	3 SETS
15 REPS	10 REPS
30-SECOND REST	30-SECOND REST
BETWEEN SETS	BETWEEN SETS

HINTS

Keep your back upright by contracting your core muscles. Do not round your lower back. • Complete the full range of motion, from the arm fully extended, to holding the dumbbell at shoulder level, and back again. • Start with your feet shoulder-width apart. To make it more challenging, bring your feet closer together.

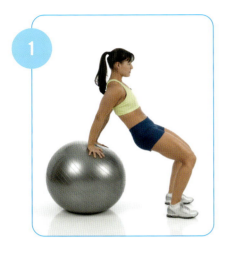
WORKOUT 1: Dips with Hands on Ball

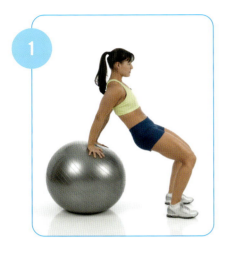

1

- With the ball behind you, place your hands on top of it, keeping your arms straight and your feet flat on the floor.

- Bend your knees slightly.

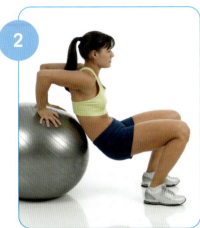

2

- Lower your body toward the floor by bending your elbows and dipping until your lower back touches the ball.

- Push up against the ball until your arms are straight again in the starting position.

- Keep your feet flat on the floor throughout the movement.

Intensity

Weight Loss	Toning
2 SETS	3 SETS
15 REPS	10 REPS
30-SECOND REST	30-SECOND REST
BETWEEN SETS	BETWEEN SETS

HINTS

You can position the ball against a wall to steady it. • Do not sit on the ball in the down position; barely touch the ball with your lower back. • To increase the difficulty, straighten your legs and place your heels on the floor. • Keep your head up and look straight ahead.

WORKOUT 1: Weighted Crunch

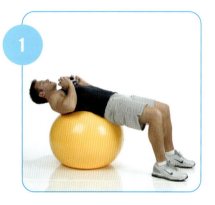

- Lie across the ball with your back in a reverse bridge position, centering the ball in your mid-back.

- Keep your head and neck off the ball.

- Hold a dumbbell in both hands under your chin and close to your chest.

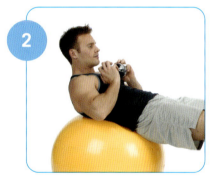

- Lift your head and shoulders up and away from the ball, contracting your abdominals.

- Roll your upper body back over the ball, returning to the starting position. Hold the dumbbell in the same position throughout the exercise.

Intensity

Weight Loss	Toning
2 SETS	3 SETS
15 REPS	10 REPS
30-SECOND REST	30-SECOND REST
BETWEEN SETS	BETWEEN SETS

HINTS

Control the movement through your midsection, and avoid jerky movements. • Keep the weight close to your chest, holding it in your hands. • Lift only your head and shoulders, not your whole back. • Start with your feet shoulder-width apart. To make it more challenging, bring your feet closer together.

WORKOUT 1: Crunch with Rotation

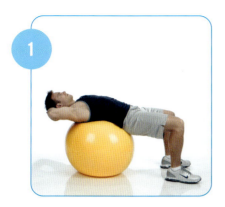

- Lie with your back on the ball in a reverse bridge position with the ball centered at your mid-back.

- Keep your head and neck off the ball and your feet flat on the floor.

- Place your hands at the sides of your head.

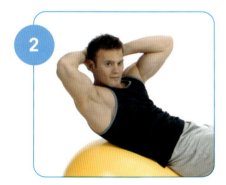

- Lift your head and shoulders up and away from the ball, and rotate them to one side by contracting your abdominals and twisting through your midsection.

- Twist back to the center and roll your upper body back over the ball, returning to the starting position.

Intensity

Weight Loss	Toning
2 SETS	3 SETS
15 REPS	10 REPS
30-SECOND REST	30-SECOND REST
BETWEEN SETS	BETWEEN SETS

HINTS

Control the movement through your midsection to avoid jerky movements. • Do not use your hands to pull your head and neck up. • Lift just your head and shoulders off the ball. • Start with your feet shoulder-width apart. To make it more challenging, bring your feet closer together.

WORKOUT 1: Front Bridge with Elbows on Ball

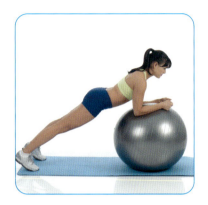

- Place your forearms on the ball and extend your legs with both feet on the floor.

- The ball should be directly under your chest, and your body should be straight.

- Hold this position for 10 seconds, then lower your body to lie on the ball.

Intensity

Weight Loss	Toning
2 SETS	3 SETS
15 REPS	10 REPS
30-SECOND REST	30-SECOND REST
BETWEEN SETS	BETWEEN SETS

HINTS

Start in a kneeling position with your elbows on the ball. Raise your hips and hold your torso in this position throughout the exercise. • Keep your forearms on top of the ball. • Start with your feet hip-width apart.

WORKOUT 1: Standing Hamstring Stretch

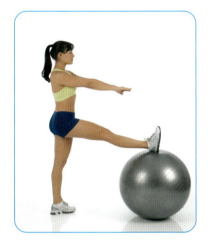

- Stand with one heel on the ball in front of you.

- Stretch your arms in front of you, and gently lean forward at the waist, stretching toward your foot.

Intensity

HOLD FOR 10 SECONDS

REPEAT 3 TIMES WITH EACH LEG

WORKOUT 1: Lying Quadriceps Stretch

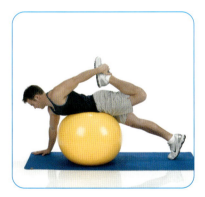

- Lie face down, centered over the ball. Position both hands and feet on the floor.

- Raise one leg, bending at the knee, and grasp your ankle with your hand.

- Pull your foot toward your buttocks.

Intensity

HOLD FOR 10 SECONDS

REPEAT 3 TIMES WITH EACH LEG

WORKOUT 1: Glute Stretch

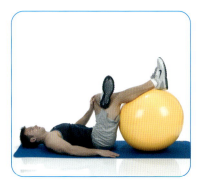

- Lie on your back on the mat. Place one leg on the ball with your knee bent.

- Place the other foot on that knee. Gently push the outside knee away from you.

Intensity

HOLD FOR 10 SECONDS
REPEAT 3 TIMES WITH EACH LEG

WORKOUT 1: Supine Chest Stretch

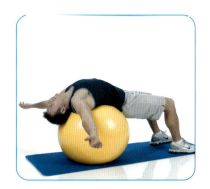

- Lie across the ball on your back with your arms stretched overhead.

- Roll back to center yourself on the ball with your head, shoulders, and arms hanging down. Lower your hands toward the floor.

Intensity

HOLD FOR 10 SECONDS
REPEAT 3 TIMES

WORKOUT 1: Spine Flexion Stretch

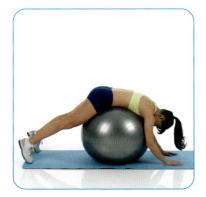

- Lie face down with the ball under your midsection.

- With your hands and feet on the floor, let your head and shoulders fall into a relaxed position.

- Allow your spine to flex as you gently rock back and forth over the ball.

Intensity

HOLD FOR 10 SECONDS

REPEAT 3 TIMES

WORKOUT 2: Single-Leg Dead Lift with Ball to Overhead

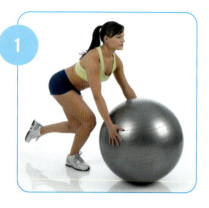

1
- Squat in front of the ball with your feet flat on the floor, your head up, and your back in a neutral position.
- Raise one foot off the floor and grasp the ball with your hands in front of you.

2
- Stand up and lift the ball overhead with your arms fully extended, keeping one foot off the floor.
- Squat down on one leg, returning to the starting position, and setting the ball on the floor.
- Repeat on your other leg.

Intensity

Weight Loss	Toning
2 SETS	**3 SETS**
15 REPS	**10 REPS**
30-SECOND REST	**30-SECOND REST**
BETWEEN SETS	**BETWEEN SETS**

HINTS

The position of your back is very important in squatting exercises. Always maintain a neutral position. Do not round your lower back or overarch it. • Keep your head up, looking straight ahead, and your shoulders back.

WORKOUT 2: Pullover

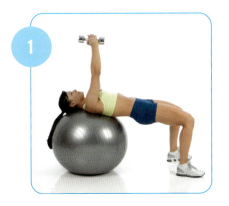

- Lie on your back in a reverse bridge position with the ball squarely between your shoulder blades and your feet flat on the floor.

- Keep your hips level with your shoulders.

- Hold one dumbbell with both hands directly over your chest with your arms fully extended upward.

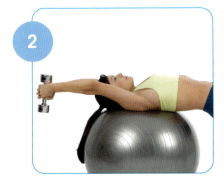

- Lower the dumbbell behind your head, keeping your arms straight behind you.

- Return the dumbbell to the starting position over your chest.

- Keep your arms completely straight throughout the exercise.

Intensity

Weight Loss	Toning
2 SETS	3 SETS
15 REPS	10 REPS
30-SECOND REST	30-SECOND REST
BETWEEN SETS	BETWEEN SETS

HINTS

Keep your hips in line with your shoulders. Do not let them sag or dip. This requires you to contract your abdominal and core muscles. • *Lower the dumbbell further behind your head once you feel comfortable with the exercise.*

WORKOUT 2: Reciprocal Wide Row

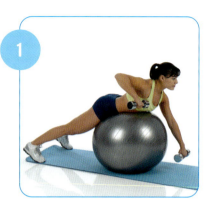

- Lie facedown with the ball centered under your mid-abdomen and your legs stretched out behind you.

- Hold a dumbbell in each hand, one at shoulder level and the other with your arm extended toward the floor.

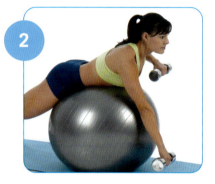

- Raise one dumbbell, drawing your shoulder blade in and bending your elbow out, while at the same time lowering the other dumbbell to the floor in a reciprocal motion.

- Alternate the movement, making sure to lower one dumbbell nearly to the floor while the other is at shoulder level.

Intensity

Weight Loss	Toning
2 SETS	3 SETS
15 REPS	10 REPS
30-SECOND REST	30-SECOND REST
BETWEEN SETS	BETWEEN SETS

HINTS

Start with your feet shoulder-width apart. To make it more challenging, bring your feet closer together. • Draw your elbows up and out to your sides, not in close. • Look down at the floor to keep your head in line with your spine. Do not raise your head as you raise the dumbbells.

WORKOUT 2: Single-Leg Prone Hamstring Curl

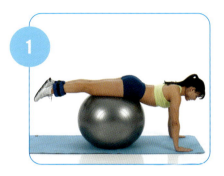

- Using ankle weights, lie facedown with the ball under your thighs.

- Place your hands on the mat directly under your shoulders with your arms fully extended.

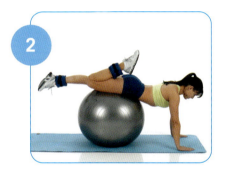

- Bending at the knee, bring one foot to your buttocks.

- Extend your leg, lowering your foot back to the starting position.

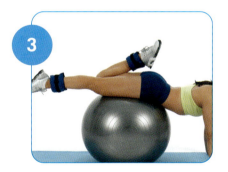

- Repeat the movement with the other foot.

Intensity

Weight Loss	Toning
2 SETS	3 SETS
15 REPS	10 REPS
30-SECOND REST	30-SECOND REST
BETWEEN SETS	BETWEEN SETS

HINTS

To maintain a neutral spine, look at the floor and do not raise your head. • Keep your arms fully extended throughout the movement. • Bring your feet in to touch your buttocks and then out to a straight-leg position.

WORKOUT 2: Lateral Raise on Single Leg

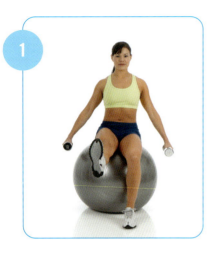

- Sit upright on the ball with one foot flat on the floor and the other leg extended in front.

- Hold a dumbbell in each hand with your palms facing in and your arms extended along your sides.

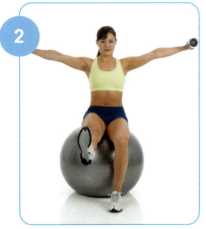

- Raise the dumbbells up and out to your sides to a position just above shoulder level, and keep your arms straight.

- Lower the dumbbells down to your sides, returning to the starting position.

Intensity

Weight Loss	Toning
2 SETS	3 SETS
15 REPS	10 REPS
30-SECOND REST	30-SECOND REST
BETWEEN SETS	BETWEEN SETS

HINTS

Keep your back upright by contracting your core muscles as you raise the dumbbells. • Avoid jerky movements. • Bend your elbows slightly to reduce stress on your shoulder joints.

WORKOUT 2: Single-Arm Twisting Curl

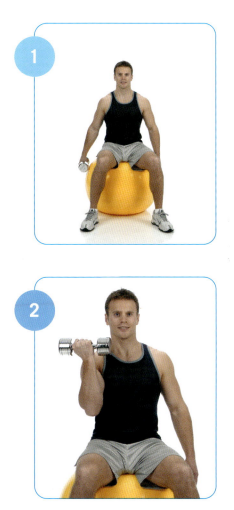

1

- Sit upright on the ball with your feet flat on the floor.

- Hold a dumbbell in one hand with your palm facing in and your arms extended along your sides.

2

- Raise the dumbbell up in front to shoulder level, bending at your elbow and twisting your wrist until your palm is facing back.

- Return the dumbbell to the starting position.

- Keep the other arm at your side throughout the entire exercise.

Intensity

Weight Loss	Toning
2 SETS	3 SETS
15 REPS	10 REPS
30-SECOND REST	30-SECOND REST
BETWEEN SETS	BETWEEN SETS

HINTS

Keep your back upright by contracting your core muscles. Do not round your lower back. • Complete the full range of motion, from the arm fully extended, to dumbbell at shoulder level, and back again. • Start with your feet shoulder-width apart. To make it more challenging, bring your feet closer together.

WORKOUT 2: Single-Arm French Press

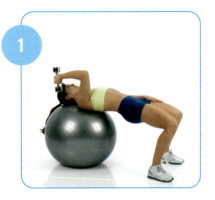

- Lie with your back on the ball in a reverse bridge position, centering the ball between your shoulder blades.

- Keep your hips level with your shoulders and your feet flat on the floor.

- Hold a dumbbell in one hand with your elbow flexed and the weight positioned at the side of your head.

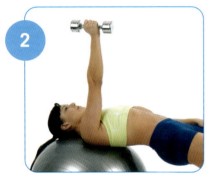

- Raise the dumbbell until your arm is straight and the weight is overhead.

- Lower the dumbbell, bending at the elbow, to return to the starting position.

- Follow through until the dumbbell is back at the side of your head.

Intensity

Weight Loss	Toning
2 SETS	3 SETS
15 REPS	10 REPS
30-SECOND REST	30-SECOND REST
BETWEEN SETS	BETWEEN SETS

HINTS

Keep your hips aligned with your shoulders. Do not let them sag or dip. This requires you to contract your abdominal and core muscles. • Be careful not to hit the back of your head with the dumbbell as you lift and lower it. • Do not allow your upper arm to move around. Keep your shoulders steady; all movement should occur at the elbow.

WORKOUT 2: Leg Raises

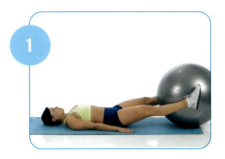

- Lie on your back on the mat with your legs straight, holding the ball between your feet.

- Place your hands by your sides.

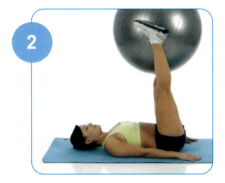

- Raise your legs, keeping them straight, and lift the ball into position over your midsection.

- Lower the ball, extending your hips to return to the starting position.

Intensity

Weight Loss	Toning
2 SETS	3 SETS
15 REPS	10 REPS
30-SECOND REST	30-SECOND REST
BETWEEN SETS	BETWEEN SETS

HINTS

Keep your head, back, and shoulders on the mat. • Keep your legs straight. • Use your hands to help stabilize yourself, pushing them into the floor when lifting your hips.

WORKOUT 2: Torso Rotation

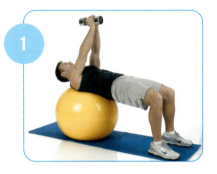

1

- Lie over the ball with your back in a reverse bridge position, centering your shoulder blades, and position your feet flat on the floor.

- Keep your hips level with your shoulders.

- Hold one dumbbell with both hands, arms fully extended upward and the dumbbell directly over your chest.

2

- Rotate your body to one side, rolling onto your shoulder and keeping your arms fully extended.

3

- Rotate 180 degrees to the other side.

Intensity

Weight Loss	Toning
2 SETS	3 SETS
15 REPS	10 REPS
30-SECOND REST	30-SECOND REST
BETWEEN SETS	BETWEEN SETS

HINTS

Keep your hips in line with your shoulders. Do not let them sag or dip. This requires you to contract your abdominal and core muscles.

WORKOUT 2: Kneeling Back Extension

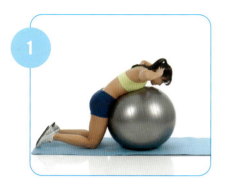

- Kneeling on the mat, place your chest on the ball and your hands at the sides of your head.

- Let your head and shoulders drape over the ball.

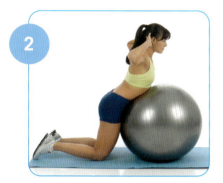

- Lift your chest up off the ball, extending your back until your upper body is straight.

- Keep your hands at the sides of your head, and return to the starting position.

Intensity

Weight Loss	Toning
2 SETS	3 SETS
15 REPS	10 REPS
30-SECOND REST	30-SECOND REST
BETWEEN SETS	BETWEEN SETS

HINTS

Lift only your head and shoulders, not your whole upper body. • *Your upper body should be straight at the top of the movement.* • *Do not overarch your lower back.*

WORKOUT 2: Lying Hamstring Stretch

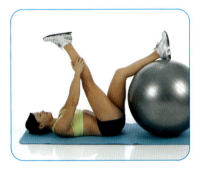

• Lie with your back on the mat. Place one leg on the ball with your knee bent.

• Keep the other leg straight and clasp your hands behind your calf.

• Slowly pull the straight leg toward your head.

Intensity

HOLD FOR 10 SECONDS
REPEAT 3 TIMES WITH EACH LEG

WORKOUT 2: Standing Quadriceps Stretch

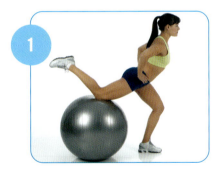

• Stand with one knee on the ball and the other foot in front.

• Gently shift your body weight forward, pushing your knee into the ball.

• For a more intense stretch, grasp the ankle of the leg on the ball and pull it toward your buttocks.

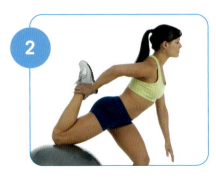

Intensity

HOLD FOR 10 SECONDS
REPEAT 3 TIMES WITH EACH LEG

WORKOUT 2: Lying Hip Adductor Stretch

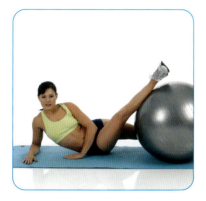

- Lie on your side with your lower leg on the ball and the other leg behind it.

- Push down on the ball with your leg and lift your upper body off the mat.

Intensity

HOLD FOR 10 SECONDS

REPEAT 3 TIMES WITH EACH LEG

WORKOUT 2: Upper Back Stretch

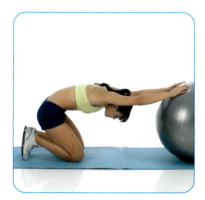

- Kneel on the floor with your hands on top of the ball held out at arms' length.

- Lower your head between your shoulders and arch your back.

- Sit back on your heels.

Intensity

HOLD FOR 10 SECONDS

REPEAT 3 TIMES

WORKOUT 2: Shoulder Stretch

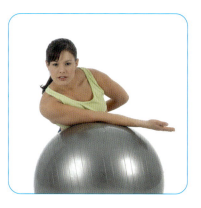

- Kneel on the floor with the ball in front of you and one arm resting on top of it.

- Relax your upper body toward the ball as you feel a stretch along the back of your shoulder.

Intensity

HOLD FOR 10 SECONDS
REPEAT 3 TIMES WITH EACH ARM

WORKOUT 3: Lunge with Ball Overhead

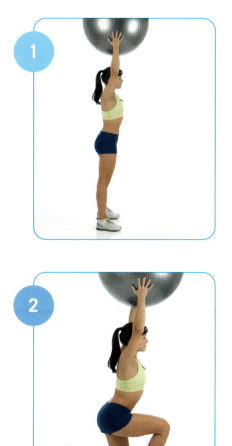

• Stand upright with your arms extended, holding the ball overhead.

• Step forward and drop your back knee toward the floor, bending at the hip and knee.

• Lean slightly forward, keeping all your weight on the front foot, still holding the ball overhead.

• Push off with the front foot to return to the starting position, and repeat with your other leg.

Intensity

Weight Loss	Toning
2 SETS	3 SETS
15 REPS	10 REPS
30-SECOND REST	30-SECOND REST
BETWEEN SETS	BETWEEN SETS

HINTS

The position of your back is very important in squatting exercises. Always maintain a neutral position, neither rounding your lower back nor overarching it. • Keep your head up, looking straight ahead with your shoulders back. • Place your weight over the leg you step onto and push off this leg to return to the central position.

WORKOUT 3: Reciprocal Chest Press

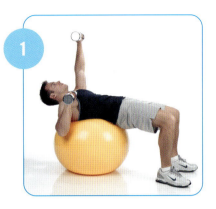

- Lie over the ball in a reverse bridge position with it centered between your shoulder blades.

- Keep your hips level with your shoulders.

- Hold a dumbbell in each hand: one at shoulder level and the other at the end of your fully extended arm.

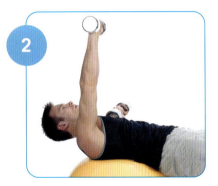

- Press one dumbbell up as you lower the other in a reciprocal motion.

- Return to your starting position, making sure to follow through until one dumbbell is at shoulder level and the other is straight overhead.

Intensity

Weight Loss	Toning
2 SETS	3 SETS
15 REPS	10 REPS
30-SECOND REST	30-SECOND REST
BETWEEN SETS	BETWEEN SETS

HINTS

Keep your hips in line with your shoulders. Do not let them sag or dip. This requires you to contract the abdominal and core muscles. • *Keep the dumbbell directly over your chest throughout the exercise. Do not let it move outward or inward.*

WORKOUT 3: Rear Deltoid Row

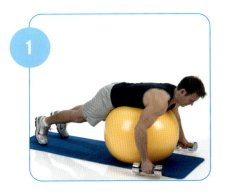

- Lie face down on the ball with it under your mid-abdomen and your legs stretched out behind you.

- Hold a dumbbell in each hand with your elbows slightly bent and palms facing each other.

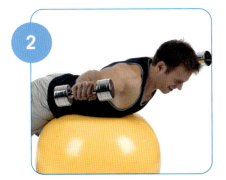

- Raise the dumbbells up and out to your sides to shoulder level.

- Keep your arms straight throughout the movement, and do not round your upper back.

Intensity

Weight Loss	Toning
2 SETS	3 SETS
15 REPS	10 REPS
30-SECOND REST	30-SECOND REST
BETWEEN SETS	BETWEEN SETS

HINTS

Start with your feet shoulder-width apart. To make it more challenging, bring your feet closer together. • Draw your arms up and out to your sides, pulling your shoulder blades together at the top. • Look down at the floor to keep your head in line with your spine. Do not lift your head as you raise the dumbbells.

WORKOUT 3: Straight-Leg Dead Lift with Ball Hold

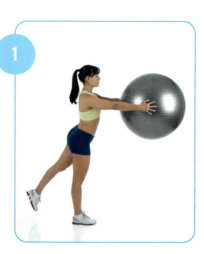

- Stand upright with your arms holding the ball, extended in front of your chest.

- Raise one foot off the floor.

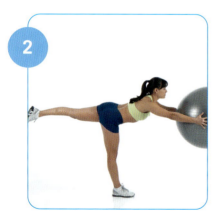

- Flex at the hip and lower the ball, keeping your arms and the standing leg straight.

- Lower to the point where your shoulders are at hip level and then return to the starting position.

- Repeat the exercise with the other leg.

Intensity

Weight Loss	Toning
2 SETS	3 SETS
15 REPS	10 REPS
30-SECOND REST	30-SECOND REST
BETWEEN SETS	BETWEEN SETS

HINTS

Keep your abdominal and core muscles activated during the movement. Do not round your lower back. •
Keep your standing leg straight throughout the exercise. A slight bend at the knee may help if you have flexibility limitations.

WORKOUT 3: Reciprocal Front Raise

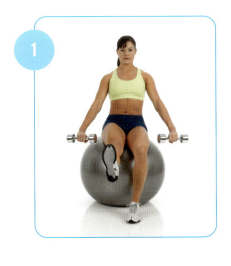

- Sit upright on the ball with one foot flat on the floor and the opposite leg extended out in front.

- Hold a dumbbell in each hand, palms facing down, and extend your arms along your sides.

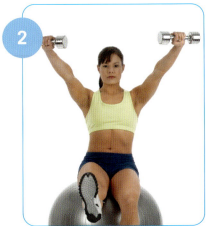

- Raise the dumbbells to just above your shoulder level and in front of you, keeping your arms straight.

- Lower the dumbbells to your sides, returning to the starting position.

- Be sure to follow through until your arms are fully extended.

Intensity

Weight Loss	Toning
2 SETS	3 SETS
15 REPS	10 REPS
30-SECOND REST	30-SECOND REST
BETWEEN SETS	BETWEEN SETS

HINTS

Keep your back upright by contracting your core muscles as you raise the dumbbells. • *Move smoothly.* • *Bend your elbows slightly to avoid stress on your shoulder joints.*

WORKOUT 3: Single-Arm Preacher Curl

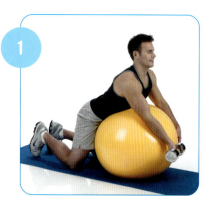

1

- Kneel on the mat with your chest and elbows on the ball, your arms fully extended over the ball, and a dumbbell in one hand.

- Keep the other hand down at the side of the ball.

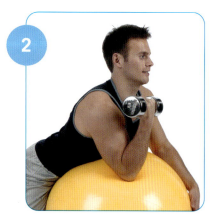

2

- Raise the dumbbell to shoulder level, bending at the elbow.

- Lower the dumbbell by extending your elbow to return to your starting position with your arm fully extended over the ball.

Intensity

Weight Loss	Toning
2 SETS	**3 SETS**
15 REPS	**10 REPS**
30-SECOND REST	**30-SECOND REST**
BETWEEN SETS	**BETWEEN SETS**

HINTS

Keep your shoulders and upper arm steady by pressing your elbows into the ball. • *Be careful not to round your upper back as you curl up.* • *Maintain a neutral spine.*

WORKOUT 3: Dips with Hands on Chair

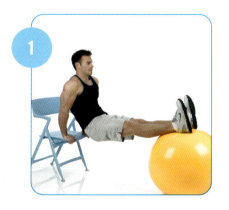

1

- With the ball in front of you, place your hands on a chair, keeping your arms straight. Then position your feet on the ball with your legs straight.

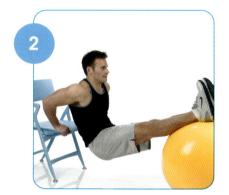

2

- Lower your body toward the floor by bending your elbows, dipping until your elbows are at shoulder level.

- Push up against the chair to the starting position where your arms are straight again.

Intensity

Weight Loss	Toning
2 SETS	**3 SETS**
15 REPS	**10 REPS**
30-SECOND REST	**30-SECOND REST**
BETWEEN SETS	**BETWEEN SETS**

HINTS

Sit on a chair with your feet on the ball. Slowly push the ball out with your feet and position your hands on the edge of the chair. Choose a steady chair that can hold your weight at the edge of its seat. • Keep your head up and look straight ahead to maintain a neutral back position. • Lower your elbows below shoulder level once you feel comfortable with the position.

WORKOUT 3: Crunch on Ball

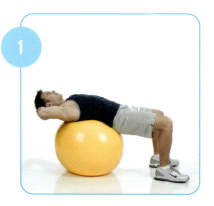

- Lie with your back on the ball in a reverse bridge position with the ball centered in your mid-back.

- Keep your head and neck off the ball and your feet flat on the floor.

- Place your hands at the sides of your head.

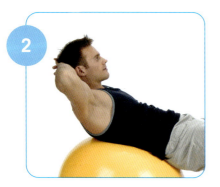

- Lift your head and shoulders up and away from the ball, contracting your abdominals.

- Roll your upper body back over the ball, returning to the starting position.

Intensity

Weight Loss	Toning
2 SETS	3 SETS
15 REPS	10 REPS
30-SECOND REST	30-SECOND REST
BETWEEN SETS	BETWEEN SETS

HINTS

Control the movement with your midsection, and avoid jerky movements. • Do not use your hands to pull your head and neck up. • Lift only your head and shoulders off the ball. • Start with your feet shoulder-width apart. To make it more challenging, bring your feet closer together.

WORKOUT 3: Lateral Bridge

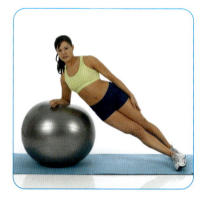

- Lie on one side with your forearm on the ball and your legs stretched out.

- Place your other arm on your side.

- Raise your hips off the ball; hold this position for 10 seconds, then lower your hips back down to the ball.

- Repeat to complete your reps, then switch sides.

Intensity

Weight Loss	Toning
2 SETS	3 SETS
15 REPS	10 REPS
30-SECOND REST	30-SECOND REST
BETWEEN SETS	BETWEEN SETS

HINTS

Start by lying on your side on the ball. Raise your hips off the ball and hold the position. • Do not let your hips sag or dip. This requires you to contract your abdominal and core muscles. • Keep your upper body aligned with your hips. Do not allow your shoulders to fall forward. • Look straight ahead to maintain a neutral spine.

WORKOUT 3: Alternating Arm and Leg Extension

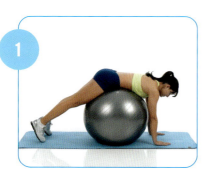

1

• Lie facedown with the ball under your abdomen and both hands and feet touching the floor.

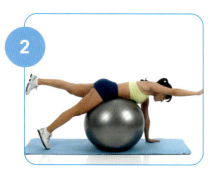

2

• Raise one arm and the opposite leg off the floor, keeping them straight.

• Lower your arm and leg back to the starting position.

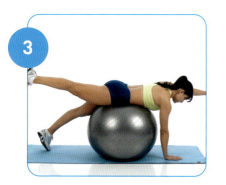

3

• Repeat with the other arm and its opposite leg.

Intensity

Weight Loss	Toning
2 SETS	**3 SETS**
15 REPS	**10 REPS**
30-SECOND REST	**30-SECOND REST**
BETWEEN SETS	**BETWEEN SETS**

HINTS

Keep the ball under your abdomen to maintain balance. • *Raise the arm and leg in line with your hips and shoulders.* • *You should feel as if you are stretching out and lengthening your spine.*

WORKOUT 3: Standing Hamstring Stretch

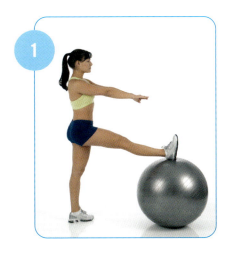

• Stand with one heel on the ball in front of you.

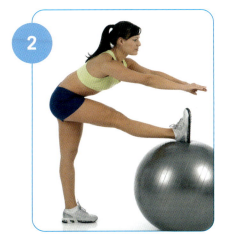

• Stretch your arms out in front of you, and gently lean forward at the waist, stretching toward your foot.

Intensity

HOLD FOR 10 SECONDS
REPEAT 3 TIMES WITH EACH LEG

WORKOUT 3: Hip Flexor Stretch

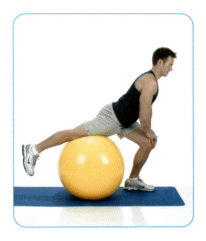

- Stand over the ball with one leg in front and the other behind you.

- Shift your weight forward, opening the hip joint of your back leg.

Intensity

HOLD FOR 10 SECONDS
REPEAT 3 TIMES WITH EACH LEG

WORKOUT 3: Lying Hip Abductor Stretch

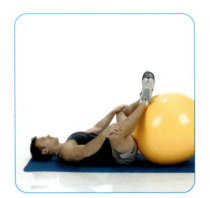

- Lie with your back on the mat and the ball in front of you.

- Place your ankles on the ball with your heels together.

- Gently push your knees away from your body.

Intensity

HOLD FOR 10 SECONDS
REPEAT 3 TIMES

WORKOUT 3: One-Sided Chest Stretch

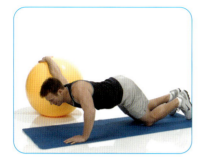

- Kneel on all fours with the ball at one side.

- Place your hand on top of the ball with one arm extended.

- Lower your body into a stretch across your upper chest.

Intensity

HOLD FOR 10 SECONDS
REPEAT 3 TIMES WITH EACH ARM

WORKOUT 3: Lateral Stretch

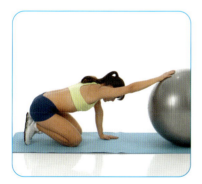

- Kneel on the floor with one hand on top of the ball held at arms' length.

- Keep your head down and look at the floor. Sit back on your heels.

- Lower your shoulder toward the floor until you feel the stretch along the side of your back.

Intensity

HOLD FOR 10 SECONDS
REPEAT 3 TIMES WITH EACH ARM

WORKOUT 4: **Single-Leg Squat to Ball**

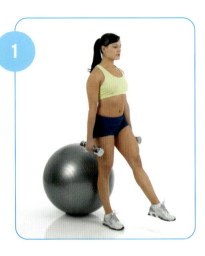

1

- Start with the ball on the floor behind you.

- Place feet facing forward, hip-width apart, and lift your leg to raise one foot off the floor.

- Hold a dumbbell in each hand.

2

- Lower your body to the ball until you just touch it, keeping one foot in the air and the leg out in front.

- Keep your back in a neutral position.

- Push through the standing foot to return to the starting position.

Intensity

Weight Loss	Toning
2 SETS	3 SETS
15 REPS	10 REPS
30-SECOND REST	30-SECOND REST
BETWEEN SETS	BETWEEN SETS

HINTS

The position of your back is very important when doing squatting exercises. Always maintain a neutral position. Do not round your lower back or overarch it. • Keep your head up, looking straight ahead, and keep your shoulders back. • Position the ball against a wall so it will not shift around as you move down and up.

WORKOUT 4: Incline Chest Press

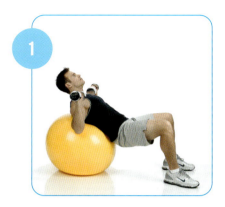

- Lie with your back on the ball in a reverse bridge position with the ball squarely between your shoulder blades.

- Drop your hips so your back is on the ball and your body is at a 45-degree angle, with your feet flat on the floor.

- Hold a dumbbell in each hand at shoulder level.

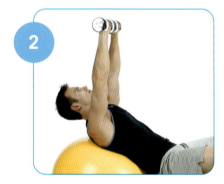

- Lift the dumbbells until your arms are straight, and the dumbbells are directly over your upper chest.

- Lower the dumbbells by bending your elbows to return to the starting position, with dumbbells at shoulder level.

Intensity

Weight Loss	Toning
2 SETS	3 SETS
15 REPS	10 REPS
30-SECOND REST	30-SECOND REST
BETWEEN SETS	BETWEEN SETS

HINTS

Although your hips and back are on the ball, you must keep your abdominal muscles contracted for stability. • *Hold the dumbbells directly over your chest. Do not let them move outward or inward.* • *Start with your feet shoulder-width apart. To make it more challenging, bring your feet closer together.*

WORKOUT 4: Reciprocal Close Row

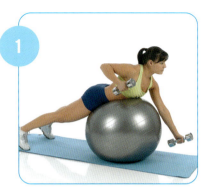

- Lie facedown with the ball under your mid-abdomen and your legs stretched out behind you.

- Hold a dumbbell in each hand with palms facing in, one at shoulder level and the other with your arm extended toward the floor.

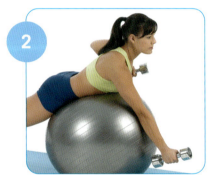

- Raise one dumbbell, drawing your shoulder blade in and bending your elbow, while at the same time lowering the other dumbbell to the floor.

- Alternate the movement, lowering one dumbbell nearly to the floor while the other is close to chest height.

Intensity

Weight Loss	Toning
2 SETS	3 SETS
15 REPS	10 REPS
30-SECOND REST	30-SECOND REST
BETWEEN SETS	BETWEEN SETS

HINTS

Start with your feet shoulder-width apart. To make it more challenging, bring your feet closer together. • *Draw up your elbows by your sides, not outward.* • *Look at the floor to keep your head aligned with your spine. Do not raise your head as you raise the dumbbells.*

WORKOUT 4: Lying Leg Extension

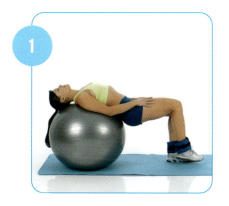

- Attach a weight to each ankle.

- Lie on the ball with your back in a reverse bridge position. Keep the ball between your shoulder blades.

- Keep one foot elevated about six inches off the floor.

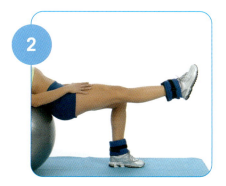

- Extend the elevated knee until your leg is straight in front.

- Lower your leg to the starting position, bending at the knee.

Intensity

Weight Loss	Toning
2 SETS	3 SETS
15 REPS	10 REPS
30-SECOND REST	30-SECOND REST
BETWEEN SETS	BETWEEN SETS

HINTS

Keep your hips in line with your shoulders. Do not let them sag or dip. This requires you to contract your abdominal and core muscles. • Place your hands on your hips. • Keep your head and shoulders on the ball throughout the exercise.

WORKOUT 4: Chest Fly

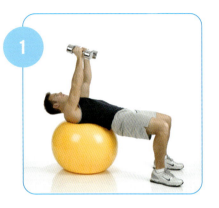

- Lie with your back in a reverse bridge position, with the ball between your shoulder blades.

- Keep your hips level with your shoulders.

- Hold a dumbbell in each hand with both arms fully extended overhead and your palms facing in.

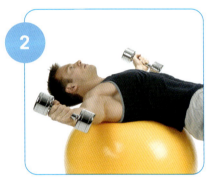

- Lower the dumbbells to the sides and down to shoulder level.

- Return to the starting position, with the dumbbells fully extended overhead.

- Keep a slight bend in your elbows throughout the movement.

Intensity

Weight Loss	Toning
2 SETS	3 SETS
15 REPS	10 REPS
30-SECOND REST	30-SECOND REST
BETWEEN SETS	BETWEEN SETS

HINTS

Keep your hips in line with your shoulders. Do not let them sag or dip. This requires you to contract the abdominals and core muscles. • Bend your elbows slightly to reduce stress on your shoulder joints. • Start with your feet shoulder-width apart. To make it more challenging, bring your feet closer together.

WORKOUT 4: Reciprocal Overhead Press

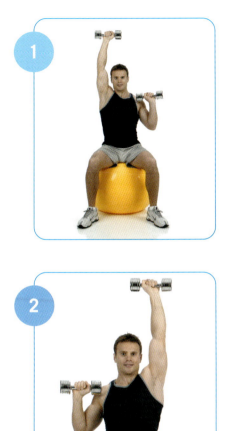

- Sit upright on the ball with your feet flat on the floor.

- Hold a dumbbell in each hand: one at shoulder level and the other overhead with your arm fully extended.

- Push up one dumbbell as you lower the other in a reciprocal motion.

- Lower the dumbbell by bending your elbow to return it to shoulder level as you press the other dumbbell back to the straight-arm position.

Intensity

Weight Loss	Toning
2 SETS	3 SETS
15 REPS	10 REPS
30-SECOND REST	30-SECOND REST
BETWEEN SETS	BETWEEN SETS

HINTS

Keep your back upright by contracting your core muscles as you push the dumbbells overhead. Do not round your lower back. • Move both dumbbells at the same time in a smooth reciprocal motion. • Start with your feet shoulder-width apart. To make it more challenging, bring your feet closer together.

WORKOUT 4: Reciprocal Hammer Curl

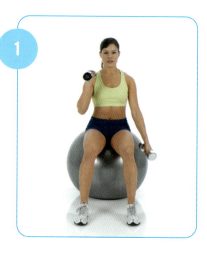

1

- Sit upright on the ball with your feet flat on the floor.
- Hold a dumbbell in each hand with your palms facing in.
- Start with one at shoulder level and the other fully extended along your side.

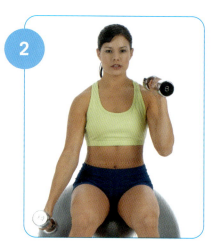

2

- Raise one dumbbell to shoulder level as you lower the other to your side in a reciprocal motion.
- Return the dumbbells to the starting positions, so that one dumbbell is at shoulder level and the other is extended by your side.

Intensity

Weight Loss	Toning
2 SETS	**3 SETS**
15 REPS	**10 REPS**
30-SECOND REST	**30-SECOND REST**
BETWEEN SETS	**BETWEEN SETS**

HINTS

Contract your core muscles to keep your back upright. Do not round your lower back. • Complete the full range of motion, from arms fully extended, to dumbbells at shoulder level, and back again. • Start with your feet shoulder-width apart. To make it more challenging, bring your feet closer together.

WORKOUT 4: Kneeling Triceps Extension

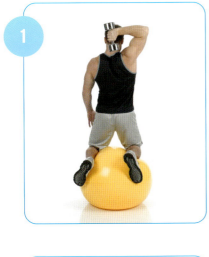

- Kneel upright on the ball.
- Hold a dumbbell behind your head with one hand, bending your elbow.

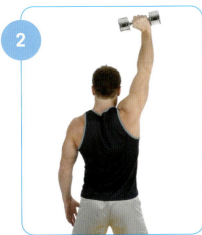

- Lift the dumbbell, extending your elbow and straightening your arm directly overhead.
- Lower the dumbbell to the starting position behind your head.

Intensity

Weight Loss	Toning
2 SETS	3 SETS
15 REPS	10 REPS
30-SECOND REST	30-SECOND REST
BETWEEN SETS	BETWEEN SETS

HINTS

Practice kneeling on the ball before attempting any exercise using weights. • Be careful not to hit your head with the dumbbell as you lift and lower it. • Do not allow your upper arm to move around. Keep your shoulder steady. All movement should be at the elbow.

WORKOUT 4: Single-Arm Lateral Raise

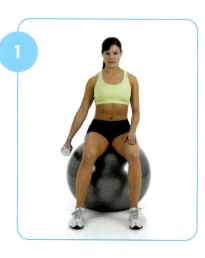

- Sit upright on the ball with your feet flat on the floor.

- Hold a dumbbell with one hand, with your palm facing in and your arm extended along your side.

- Keep the other hand at your side or place on your knee.

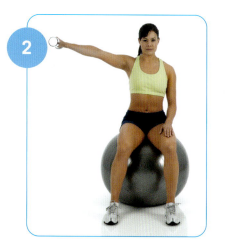

- Raise the dumbbell up and out to just above shoulder level, keeping this arm straight, and the other arm by your side.

- Lower the dumbbell to the starting position.

Intensity

Weight Loss	Toning
2 SETS	3 SETS
15 REPS	10 REPS
30-SECOND REST	30-SECOND REST
BETWEEN SETS	BETWEEN SETS

HINTS

Keep your back upright by contracting your core muscles as you lift the dumbbells. • Avoid jerky movements. • Bend your elbow slightly to reduce stress on your shoulder joint. • Start with your feet shoulder-width apart. To make it more challenging, bring your feet closer together.

WORKOUT 4: Arm to Leg Transfer

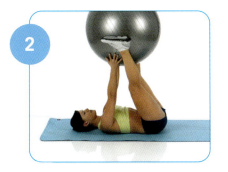

• Lie on your back on the mat with your legs straight and your arms overhead, holding the ball with your hands. Hold arms and legs slightly off the ground.

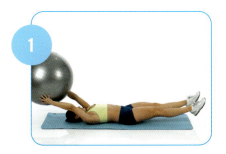

• Simultaneously lift your arms and legs straight up, holding the ball over your midsection.

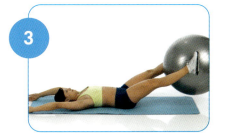

• Transfer the ball from your hands to your feet. Lower both arms and legs, returning to the starting position with the ball now between your feet.

• Reverse the movement.

Intensity

Weight Loss	Toning
2 SETS	3 SETS
15 REPS	10 REPS
30-SECOND REST	30-SECOND REST
BETWEEN SETS	BETWEEN SETS

HINTS

Keep your arms and legs straight throughout the exercise. • If you like, set your feet on the mat at the end of each repetition. To increase the difficulty, keep your feet off the mat at all times.

WORKOUT 4: Single-Leg Reverse Bridge

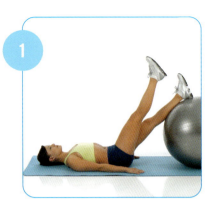

- Lie on your back on the mat with both heels on the ball and legs extended.

- Place your hands by your sides and raise one foot off the ball.

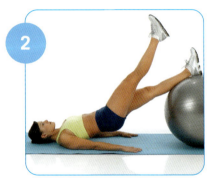

- Raise your hips off the mat by contracting your abdominals, and hold this position.

- Lower your hips to the mat, returning to the starting position.

- Repeat for each repetition and then switch legs.

Intensity

Weight Loss	Toning
2 SETS	3 SETS
15 REPS	10 REPS
30-SECOND REST	30-SECOND REST
BETWEEN SETS	BETWEEN SETS

HINTS

Keep your core and abdominal muscles contracted to maintain a neutral spinal position. • *Use your hands to help stabilize yourself. Push them into the floor while raising your hips.* • *Only your head, upper back, and shoulders should contact the mat at the top position.*

WORKOUT 4: Scissors

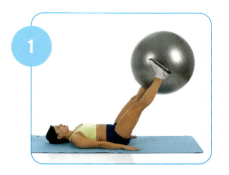

- Lie back on the mat with the ball between your feet and your legs straight at a 45-degree angle to the floor.

- Place your hands at your sides.

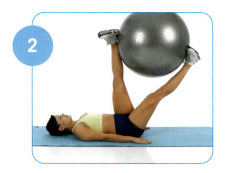

- Roll the ball between your feet, twisting your legs and lower body to one side.

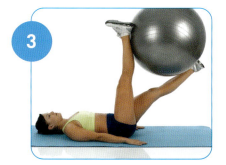

- Roll the ball to the opposite direction, twisting to the other side.

Intensity

Weight Loss	Toning
2 SETS	3 SETS
15 REPS	10 REPS
30-SECOND REST	30-SECOND REST
BETWEEN SETS	BETWEEN SETS

HINTS

Keep your head, back, and shoulders on the mat. • *Keep your legs straight throughout the exercise.* • *Use your hands to help stabilize yourself.*

WORKOUT 4: Lying Hamstring Stretch

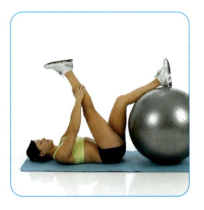

- Lie on your back on the mat with the ball in front of you. Place one leg on the ball with your knee bent.

- Keep the other leg straight, and clasp your hands behind your calf.

- Slowly pull the straight leg toward your head.

Intensity

HOLD FOR 10 SECONDS
REPEAT 3 TIMES WITH EACH LEG

WORKOUT 4: Glute Stretch

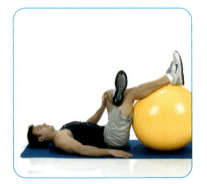

- Lie on your back on the mat. Place one leg on the ball with your knee bent.

- Place the other foot across that knee. Gently push the outside knee away from you.

Intensity

HOLD FOR 10 SECONDS
REPEAT 3 TIMES WITH EACH LEG

WORKOUT 4: Standing Hip Abductor Stretch

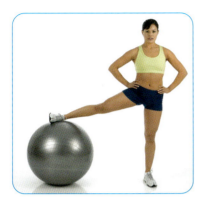

- Stand with the inside ankle of one leg positioned on the ball.

- Slowly lower your body, stretching the inside of the leg on the ball.

Intensity

HOLD FOR 10 SECONDS

REPEAT 3 TIMES WITH EACH LEG

WORKOUT 4: Lateral Spine Flexion Stretch

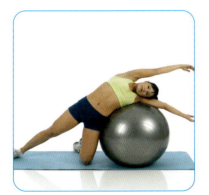

- Kneel beside the ball with your arms extended overhead.

- Lean over the ball as you extend your far leg straight.

Intensity

HOLD FOR 10 SECONDS

REPEAT 3 TIMES ON EACH SIDE

WORKOUT 4: Triceps Stretch

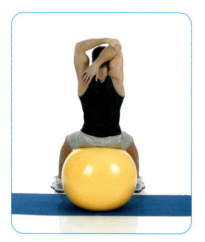

- Sit upright on the ball with one arm held behind your head, bent at the elbow.

- Place the other hand on that elbow and slowly pull it across to the middle of your back.

Intensity

HOLD FOR 10 SECONDS
REPEAT 3 TIMES WITH EACH ARM

WORKOUT 1: Lunge with Ball Overhead

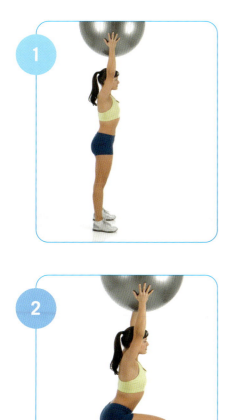

• Stand upright with your arms extended overhead holding the ball.

• Step forward and drop your back knee down toward the floor, bending at the hip and knee.

• Lean slightly forward, keeping all your weight on your front foot and the ball overhead.

• Push off your front foot to return to the starting position. Repeat with the other leg.

Intensity

Weight Loss	Toning
3 SETS	**3 SETS**
15 REPS	**8 REPS**
30-SECOND REST	**30-SECOND REST**
BETWEEN SETS	**BETWEEN SETS**

HINTS

The position of your back is very important in performing squatting exercises. Always maintain a neutral position. Do not round your lower back or overarch it. • Keep your head up, looking straight ahead, with your shoulders back, throughout the entire movement. • Place your weight over the leg you step onto, and push off this leg to return to the middle stance.

WORKOUT 1: Push-Up with Hands on Ball

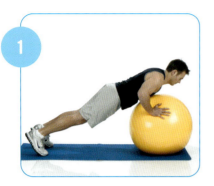

- Start with your hands on the ball directly over your shoulders and your legs extended with your feet on the floor.

- Your chest should nearly touch the ball with your body fully extended.

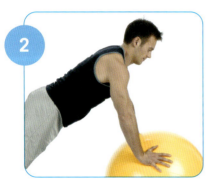

- Push up and away from the ball, extending your arms fully.

- Lower your body back to the ball, returning to the starting position. Again, your chest should nearly touch the ball.

Intensity

Weight Loss	Toning
3 SETS	3 SETS
15 REPS	8 REPS
30-SECOND REST	30-SECOND REST
BETWEEN SETS	BETWEEN SETS

HINTS

Start in a kneeling position with your hands on the ball. Raise your hips and hold your torso in this position throughout the exercise. • Move all the way up and all the way down, until your chest is nearly touching the ball. • Start with your feet hip-width apart.

WORKOUT 1: Single-Arm Close Row on Single Leg

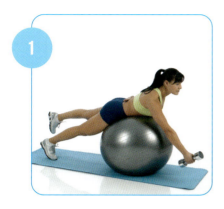

- Lie facedown with the ball under your mid-abdomen, your legs stretched out behind you, and one foot raised about 12 inches off the floor.

- In the hand opposite to your raised leg, hold a dumbbell with your elbow slightly bent and your palm facing in.

- Place the other hand behind your back.

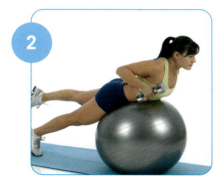

- Raise the dumbbell, drawing your shoulder blade in and bending your elbow.

- Lower the dumbbell back toward the floor, extending at the elbow.

- Keep one foot off the floor throughout the exercise.

Intensity

Weight Loss	Toning
3 SETS	**3 SETS**
15 REPS	**8 REPS**
30-SECOND REST	**30-SECOND REST**
BETWEEN SETS	**BETWEEN SETS**

HINTS

Draw your elbow up by your side, not outward. • Look down at the floor to keep your head in line with your spine. Do not raise your head as you raise the dumbbell. • Keep your leg about 12 inches off the floor throughout the exercise.

WORKOUT 1: Straight-Leg Dead Lift with Ball Hold

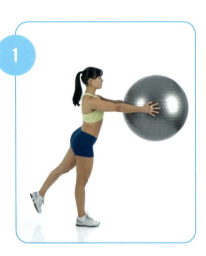

1

- Stand upright with your arms extended in front of your chest, holding the ball.

- Raise one foot off the floor.

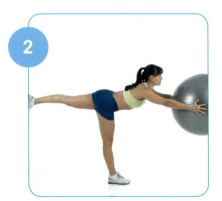

2

- Flexing at your hip, lower the ball, keeping your arms and the standing leg straight.

- Lower to the point where your shoulders are hip level, then return to the starting position.

- Repeat and switch legs.

Intensity

Weight Loss	Toning
3 SETS	3 SETS
15 REPS	8 REPS
30-SECOND REST	30-SECOND REST
BETWEEN SETS	BETWEEN SETS

HINTS

Keep your abdominal and core muscles activated during the exercise. Do not round your lower back. • *Your standing leg should remain straight throughout the exercise. A slight bend at the knee may help people with flexibility limitations.*

WORKOUT 1: Kneeling Overhead Press

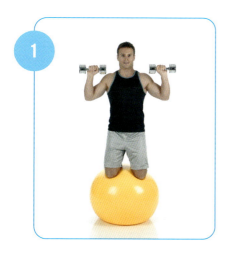

- Kneel upright on the ball, holding a dumbbell in each hand at shoulder level with your palms facing forward.

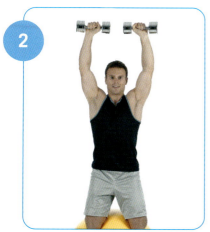

- Lift the dumbbells overhead, extending your arms.
- Lower the dumbbells to the starting position. Be sure to lower the dumbbells to shoulder level.

Intensity

Weight Loss	Toning
3 SETS	**3 SETS**
15 REPS	**8 REPS**
30-SECOND REST	**30-SECOND REST**
BETWEEN SETS	**BETWEEN SETS**

HINTS

Practice kneeling on the ball before you attempt any exercise with weights. • *Complete the full range of motion, from shoulder level, to arms fully extended overhead, and back again.*

WORKOUT 1: Single-Arm Chest Fly

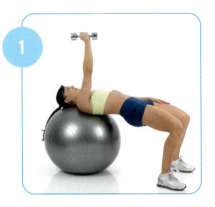

1

- Lie on your back in a reverse bridge position with the ball squarely between your shoulder blades.

- Keep your hips level with your shoulders.

- Hold a dumbbell in one hand with your arm fully extended overhead and your palm facing in. Keep the other arm by your side.

2

- Lower the dumbbell to the side and then down to shoulder level.

- Return to the starting position with the dumbbell fully extended overhead.

- Keep a slight bend in your elbow throughout the exercise.

Intensity

Weight Loss	Toning
3 SETS	**3 SETS**
15 REPS	**8 REPS**
30-SECOND REST	**30-SECOND REST**
BETWEEN SETS	**BETWEEN SETS**

HINTS

Keep your hips aligned with your shoulders. Do not let them sag or dip. This requires you to contract your abdominal and core muscles. • Bend your elbow slightly to reduce stress on your shoulder joint. • Start with your feet shoulder-width apart. To make it more challenging, bring your feet closer together.

WORKOUT 1: Reciprocal Twisting Curl

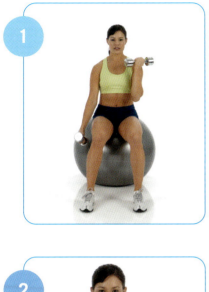

- Sit upright on the ball with your feet flat on the floor.

- Hold a dumbbell in each hand, starting with one at shoulder level, and the other with your arm fully extended at your side with your palm facing in.

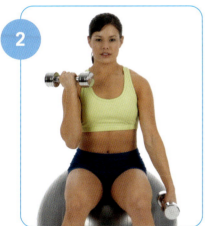

- Raise one dumbbell to shoulder level as you lower the other to your side in a reciprocal motion.

- Return the dumbbells to the starting position: one dumbbell at shoulder level and the other extended by your side.

Intensity

Weight Loss	Toning
3 SETS	3 SETS
15 REPS	8 REPS
30-SECOND REST	30-SECOND REST
BETWEEN SETS	BETWEEN SETS

HINTS

Keep your back upright by contracting your core muscles. Do not round your lower back. • Complete the full range of motion, from arms fully extended, to dumbbells at shoulder level, then back again. • Start with your feet shoulder-width apart. To make it more challenging, bring your feet closer together.

WORKOUT 1: Dips with Hands on Chair

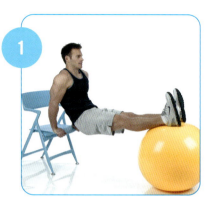

• With the ball in front of you, position your hands on a chair, keeping your arms straight. Then place your feet on the ball with your legs straight.

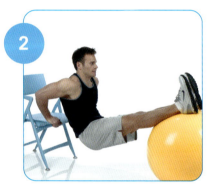

• Lower your body toward the floor, bending at the elbows, dipping until your elbows are at shoulder level.

• Push against the chair to return to the starting position where your arms are straight again.

Intensity

Weight Loss	*Toning*
3 SETS	3 SETS
15 REPS	8 REPS
30-SECOND REST	30-SECOND REST
BETWEEN SETS	BETWEEN SETS

HINTS

Start by sitting on the chair with your feet on the ball. Slowly push the ball out with your feet and position your hands on the edge of the chair. Be sure to use a sturdy chair that will support your weight. • Keep your head up, and look straight ahead to maintain a neutral back position. • Deepen the dip when you feel comfortable with the exercise.

WORKOUT 1: Hip Raises

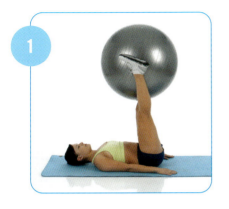

- Lie on your back on the mat with the ball between your feet and your legs straight up.

- Place your hands at your sides.

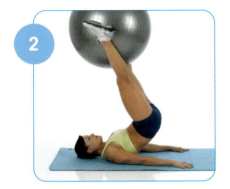

- Raise your hips and lower back off the mat, pushing the ball up.

- Return to the starting position, keeping your legs straight up.

Intensity

Weight Loss	Toning
3 SETS	**3 SETS**
15 REPS	**8 REPS**
30-SECOND REST	**30-SECOND REST**
BETWEEN SETS	**BETWEEN SETS**

HINTS

Keep your upper back and shoulders on the mat. • Do not alter your leg position. Keep your legs straight throughout the exercise. • Use your hands to help stabilize yourself, pushing them into the floor while raising your hips. At the top position, only your head, shoulders, and upper back should be in contact with the mat.

WORKOUT 1: Weighted Back Extension

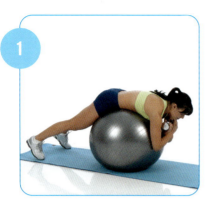

- Lie facedown with your chest on the ball and your legs extended.

- Hold a dumbbell with both hands under your chin, and let your head and shoulders drape over the ball.

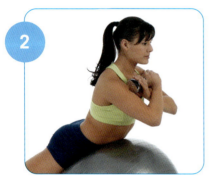

- Lift your chest off the ball, extending through your back with the weight held under your chin.

- Lower your upper body by flexing at the midsection, then returning to the starting position with your chest on the ball.

Intensity

Weight Loss	Toning
3 SETS	3 SETS
15 REPS	8 REPS
30-SECOND REST	30-SECOND REST
BETWEEN SETS	BETWEEN SETS

HINTS

Lift only your head and shoulders, not your whole upper body. • Hold your upper body straight at the top of the movement. • Do not overarch your lower back. • Push your toes into the floor to help keep you stable and prevent slipping.

WORKOUT 1: Lateral Bridge

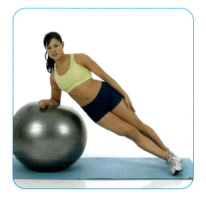

- Lie on one side with your forearm on the ball and your legs stretched out.

- Place your other arm on your side.

- Hold this position for 10 seconds then lower your hips back to the ball.

- Repeat according to the intensity level you have chosen, then switch sides.

Intensity

Weight Loss	Toning
3 SETS	3 SETS
15 REPS	8 REPS
30-SECOND REST	30-SECOND REST
BETWEEN SETS	BETWEEN SETS

HINTS

Start by lying on your side on the ball. Raise your hips off the ball and hold this position. • Do not let your hips sag or dip. Contract your abdominal and core muscles. • Keep your upper body aligned with your hips. Do not allow your shoulders to fall forward. • Look straight ahead to maintain a neutral spine.

WORKOUT 1: Wood Chops

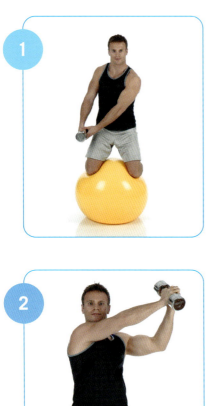

1

- Kneel on the ball, holding a dumbbell with both hands.
- Hold the dumbbell down at one side.

2

- Lift the dumbbell up and across your body, crossing to the opposite shoulder.
- Lower the dumbbell across your body to the starting position.
- Repeat on the opposite side.

Intensity

Weight Loss	Toning
3 SETS	3 SETS
15 REPS	8 REPS
30-SECOND REST	30-SECOND REST
BETWEEN SETS	BETWEEN SETS

HINTS

Practice kneeling on the ball before you attempt any exercise with weights. • Avoid jerky movements. • Follow the pattern of chopping a tree, bringing the dumbbell up and over one shoulder, then back down and across the body to the opposite side.

WORKOUT 1: Standing Hamstring Stretch

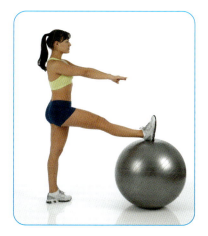

- Stand with one heel on the ball in front of you.

- Stretch your arms out in front, and gently lean forward at the waist, bringing your hands toward your foot.

Intensity

HOLD FOR 10 SECONDS
REPEAT 3 TIMES WITH EACH LEG

WORKOUT 1: Lying Quadriceps Stretch

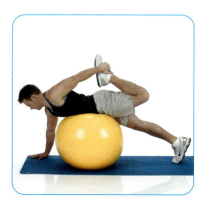

- Lie facedown with the ball under your midsection. Start with both hands and feet on the floor.

- Raise one leg, bending at the knee, and hold that ankle with your hand.

- Pull your foot toward your buttocks.

Intensity

HOLD FOR 10 SECONDS
REPEAT 3 TIMES WITH EACH LEG

WORKOUT 1: Glute Stretch

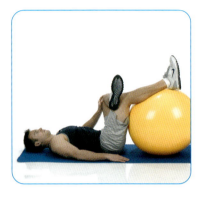

- Lie on your back on the mat. Place one leg on the ball with your knee bent.

- Position the other foot on that knee. Gently push the outside knee away from you.

Intensity

HOLD FOR 10 SECONDS
REPEAT 3 TIMES WITH EACH LEG

WORKOUT 1: Supine Chest Stretch

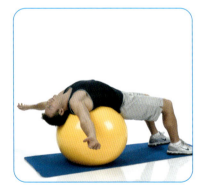

- Lie on your back over the ball with your arms stretched overhead.

- Roll back on the ball so it rests at your mid-back with your head, shoulders, and arms hanging over it. Lower your hands toward the floor.

Intensity

HOLD FOR 10 SECONDS
REPEAT 3 TIMES

WORKOUT 1: Spine Flexion Stretch

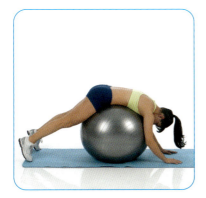

- Lie facedown with the ball under your midsection.

- Place your hands and feet on the floor, and let your head and shoulders fall forward over the ball.

- Allow your spine to flex as you stretch over the ball.

Intensity

HOLD FOR 10 SECONDS
REPEAT 3 TIMES

WORKOUT 2: Single-Leg Wall Squat

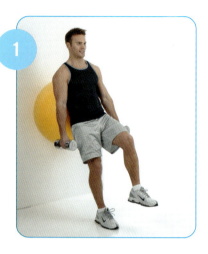

1

- Hold the ball against a wall at your lower-back level.

- Place your feet ahead of the ball, hip-width apart.

- Raise one foot off the floor. Grasp a dumbbell in each hand.

2

- Lower your body toward the floor, pushing slightly against the ball.

- Keep one foot in the air and your leg out in front.

- Squat until your thighs are parallel to the floor.

- Lift yourself to the starting position.

Intensity

Weight Loss	Toning
3 SETS	**3 SETS**
15 REPS	**8 REPS**
30-SECOND REST	**30-SECOND REST**
BETWEEN SETS	**BETWEEN SETS**

HINTS

Keep your head up and look straight ahead throughout the exercise. Do not look down at the floor or your feet. • Keep your standing foot flat on the floor with your heel down as you move up and down. • Push back against the ball throughout the exercise.

WORKOUT 2: Pullover

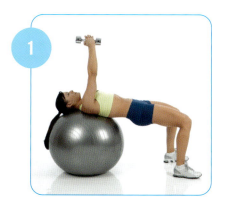

- Lie over the ball in a reverse bridge position with the ball centered between your shoulder blades and your feet flat on the floor.

- Keep your hips level with your shoulders.

- Hold a dumbbell with both hands with your arms fully extended upward and the dumbbell directly over your chest.

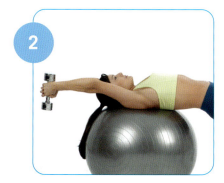

- Lower the dumbbell back behind your head, keeping your arms straight until they are directly overhead.

- Return the dumbbell to the starting position over your chest.

- Keep your arms completely straight throughout the movement.

Intensity

Weight Loss	Toning
3 SETS	3 SETS
15 REPS	8 REPS
30-SECOND REST	30-SECOND REST
BETWEEN SETS	BETWEEN SETS

HINTS

Keep your hips in line with your shoulders. Do not let them sag or dip. This requires you to contract your abdominal and core muscles. • Practice lowering the dumbbell further behind your head once you feel comfortable with the exercise.

WORKOUT 2: Wide Row on Single Leg

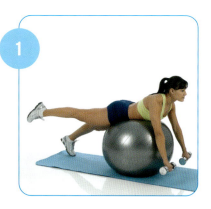

- Lie facedown with the ball under your mid-abdomen, your legs stretched out behind you, and one foot slightly off the floor.

- Hold a dumbbell in each hand with elbows slightly bent and facing out to the sides.

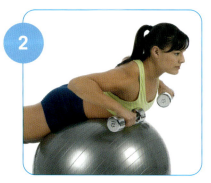

- Raise the dumbbells, drawing your shoulder blades together and bending your elbows outward.

- Lower the dumbbells back toward the floor, extending at the elbows.

- Keep one foot off the floor throughout the exercise.

Intensity

Weight Loss	Toning
3 SETS	3 SETS
15 REPS	8 REPS
30-SECOND REST	30-SECOND REST
BETWEEN SETS	BETWEEN SETS

HINTS

Draw your elbows up and out to your sides, not in close. • Look down at the floor to keep your head in line with your spine. Do not raise your head as you raise the dumbbells. • Adjust the leg held off the floor to help you maintain balance on the ball.

WORKOUT 2: Single-Leg Hamstring Curl

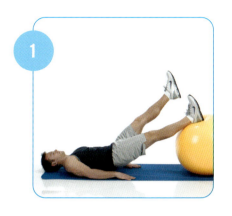

- Lie on your back on the mat with your heels on the ball and your legs extended.

- Place your hands by your sides, raise your hips off the mat, contracting your abdominals, and raise one foot off the ball, lifting your leg.

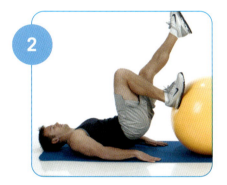

- Pull the ball towards your buttocks, bending your knee, and roll the ball from your heel to the bottom of your foot.

- Extend your leg, and return the ball to the starting position with your heel back on the ball, keeping the other foot in the air.

- Repeat the exercise and switch legs.

Intensity

Weight Loss	Toning
3 SETS	**3 SETS**
15 REPS	**8 REPS**
30-SECOND REST	**30-SECOND REST**
BETWEEN SETS	**BETWEEN SETS**

HINTS

Keep your core and abdominal muscles contracted to maintain a neutral spine throughout the exercise. • Use your hands to help stabilize yourself, pushing them into the floor when drawing your knees in. • Only your head, upper back, and shoulders should touch the mat at the top position.

WORKOUT 2: Front Raise on Single Leg

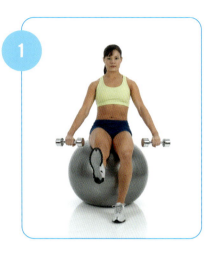

- Sit upright on the ball with one foot flat on the floor and the other leg extended in front.

- Hold a dumbbell in each hand with your palms facing backwards and your arms extended by your sides.

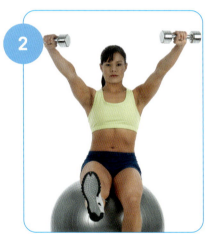

- Raise the dumbbells in front to just above your shoulder level. Keep your arms straight.

- Lower the dumbbells down to your sides, returning to the starting position.

- Lower the dumbbells until your arms are fully extended.

Intensity

Weight Loss	Toning
3 SETS	3 SETS
15 REPS	8 REPS
30-SECOND REST	30-SECOND REST
BETWEEN SETS	BETWEEN SETS

HINTS

Keep your back upright by contracting your core muscles as you raise the dumbbells. • Avoid jerky movements. • Bend your elbows slightly to reduce stress on your shoulder joints.

WORKOUT 2: Single-Arm Chest Press

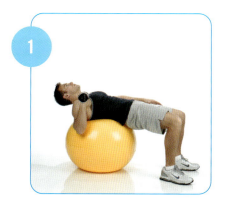

- Lie on the ball with your back in a reverse bridge position, centering the ball between your shoulder blades.

- Keep your hips level with your shoulders.

- Hold a dumbbell in one hand at shoulder level. Keep the other hand by your side.

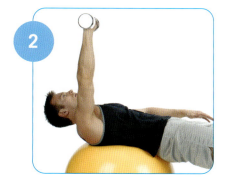

- Lift the dumbbell until your arm is straight, and the dumbbell is directly above your upper chest.

- Lower the dumbbell by bending your elbow to return to the starting position, all the way back down to shoulder level.

Intensity

Weight Loss	Toning
3 SETS	3 SETS
15 REPS	8 REPS
30-SECOND REST	30-SECOND REST
BETWEEN SETS	BETWEEN SETS

HINTS

Keep your hips in line with your shoulders. Do not let them sag or dip. This requires you to contract your abdominal and core muscles. • Hold the dumbbell directly over your chest. Do not let it move outward or inward. • Start with your feet shoulder-width apart. To make it more challenging, bring your feet closer together.

WORKOUT 2: **Kneeling Straight Curl**

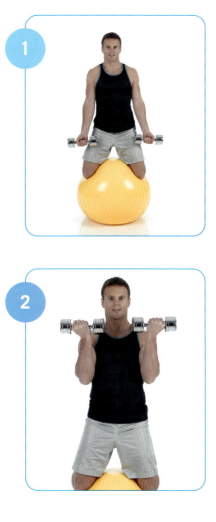

1

• Kneel upright on the ball, holding a dumbbell in each hand with your palms facing forward and your arms extended by your sides.

2

• Raise the dumbbells up in front to shoulder level, bending your elbows.

• Lower the dumbbells to the starting position at your sides.

Intensity

Weight Loss	Toning
3 SETS	**3 SETS**
15 REPS	**8 REPS**
30-SECOND REST	**30-SECOND REST**
BETWEEN SETS	**BETWEEN SETS**

HINTS

Practice kneeling on the ball before attempting any exercise with weights. • Complete the full range of motion, from arms fully extended, to dumbbells at shoulder level, and back again.

WORKOUT 2: **Single-Arm French Press**

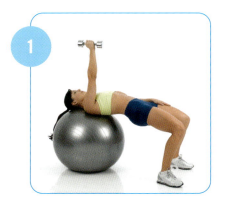

- Lie across the ball in a reverse bridge position with it centered between your shoulder blades.

- Keep your hips level with your shoulders and your feet flat on the floor.

- Hold a dumbbell in one hand with your elbow flexed, and the weight positioned at the side of your head.

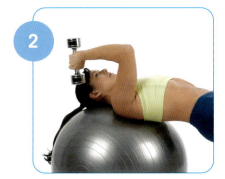

- Raise the dumbbell until your arm is straight and the weight is overhead.

- Lower the dumbbell, bending at the elbow, to return to the starting position.

- Complete the action so the dumbbell is back at the side of your head.

Intensity

Weight Loss	Toning
3 SETS	3 SETS
15 REPS	8 REPS
30-SECOND REST	30-SECOND REST
BETWEEN SETS	BETWEEN SETS

HINTS

Keep your hips in line with your shoulders. Do not let them sag or dip. This requires you to contract your abdominal and core muscles. • *Be careful not to hit the back of your head with the dumbbell as you lift and lower it.* • *Do not allow your upper arm to move. Keep your shoulder steady; the only movement is at the elbow.*

WORKOUT 2: Tuck with Side Rotation

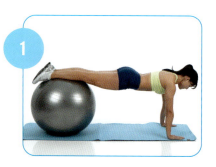

1

- Start with your hands on the mat directly under your shoulders, with your arms fully extended, and your shins on the ball.

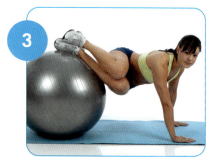

2

- Drag the ball toward your hands, bending your knees and bringing them to your chest.

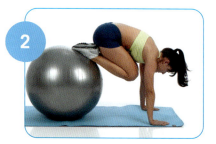

3

- Rotate your lower body to one side, bringing your knees up and to the side.

- Extend your knees and straighten your legs, returning the ball to the starting position. Repeat the exercise, rotating to the other side.

Intensity

Weight Loss	Toning
3 SETS	**3 SETS**
15 REPS	**8 REPS**
30-SECOND REST	**30-SECOND REST**
BETWEEN SETS	**BETWEEN SETS**

HINTS

Keep your hips in line with your shoulders. This requires you to contract the abdominal and core muscles.
- *Look down at the floor to maintain a neutral spine until you rotate, then turn your head to the same side.*

WORKOUT 2: Front Bridge with Hands on Ball

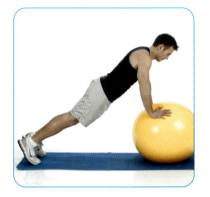

- Place your hands on the ball with your arms and legs extended and your feet on the floor hip-width apart.

- The ball should be directly under your chest. Hold your body straight.

- Hold this position for 10 seconds, then lower your body to lie on the ball.

Intensity

Weight Loss	Toning
3 SETS	3 SETS
15 REPS	8 REPS
30-SECOND REST	30-SECOND REST
BETWEEN SETS	BETWEEN SETS

HINTS

Start in a kneeling position with your hands on the ball. Raise your hips first, then straighten your torso. Keep it straight throughout the exercise. • *Keep your arms fully extended and your hands on top of the ball.*

WORKOUT 2: Arm to Leg Transfer

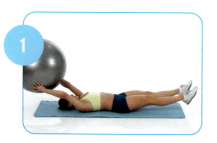

• Lie on your back on the mat with your legs straight, your arms overhead, and hold the ball in your hands.

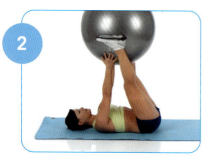

• Simultaneously, raise your arms and legs, keeping them straight to bring the ball over your midsection.

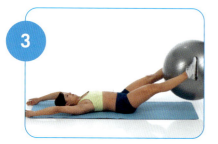

• Transfer the ball from your hands to between your feet. Lower both your arms and legs, returning to the starting position, with the ball now between your feet.

• Reverse the movement.

Intensity

Weight Loss	Toning
3 SETS	3 SETS
15 REPS	8 REPS
30-SECOND REST	30-SECOND REST
BETWEEN SETS	BETWEEN SETS

HINTS

Keep your arms and legs straight throughout the exercise. • *You may touch the mat with your feet at the end of each repetition. To increase the difficulty, hold your feet above the mat at all times.*

WORKOUT 2: Bicycle Crunch

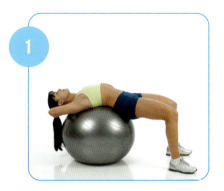

1

- Lie over the ball with your back in a reverse bridge position and the ball at your mid-back.
- Keep your head and neck off the ball.
- Place your hands at the sides of your head.

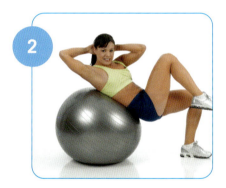

2

- Lift your head and shoulders up and away from the ball, and rotate them to one side, contracting your abdominals and twisting through your midsection.
- Raise the opposite leg off the floor, bringing your knee towards your elbow.
- Repeat this exercise on the other side.

Intensity

Weight Loss	Toning
3 SETS	3 SETS
15 REPS	8 REPS
30-SECOND REST	30-SECOND REST
BETWEEN SETS	BETWEEN SETS

HINTS

Keep your hips in line with your shoulders. Do not let them sag or dip. This requires you to contract your abdominal and core muscles. • Slide down a bit on the ball as you bring your knee to your elbow. This will help you maintain your balance. • Turn your head and shoulders as you rotate to the side.

WORKOUT 2: Lying Hamstring Stretch

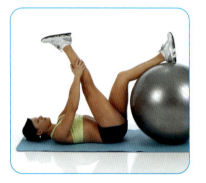

- Lie on your back on the mat. Place one leg on the ball with your knee bent.

- Keep the other leg straight, and clasp your hands behind your calf.

- Slowly pull the straight leg toward your head.

Intensity

HOLD FOR 10 SECONDS
REPEAT 3 TIMES WITH EACH LEG

WORKOUT 2: Standing Quadriceps Stretch

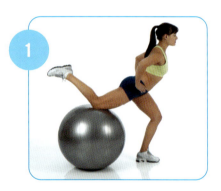

- Stand with one knee on the ball and the other foot in front.

- Gently lean forward, pushing your knee into the ball.

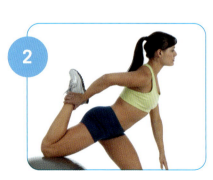

- For a more intense stretch, grasp the ankle of the leg on the ball, and pull it toward your buttocks.

Intensity

HOLD FOR 10 SECONDS
REPEAT 3 TIMES WITH EACH LEG

WORKOUT 2: Lying Hip Adductor Stretch

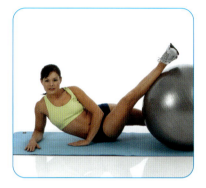

- Lie on your side with your lower leg on the ball, and the other leg behind it.

- Push on the ball with your lower leg and lift your upper body off the mat.

Intensity

HOLD FOR 10 SECONDS
REPEAT 3 TIMES WITH EACH LEG

WORKOUT 2: Upper Back Stretch

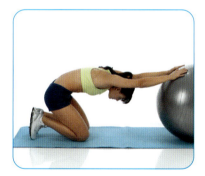

- Kneel on the floor with your hands on top of the ball, holding the ball at arm's length.

- Lower your head between your shoulders and arch your back.

- Sit back on your heels.

Intensity

HOLD FOR 10 SECONDS
REPEAT 3 TIMES

WORKOUT 2: Shoulder Stretch

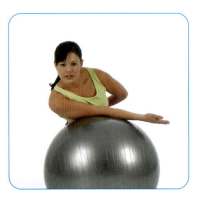

- Kneel on the floor with the ball in front of you and your upper arm resting on top of it.

- Lower your upper body toward the ball as you feel a stretch along the back of your shoulder.

Intensity

HOLD FOR 10 SECONDS
REPEAT 3 TIMES WITH EACH ARM

WORKOUT 3: Split Squat with Foot on Ball

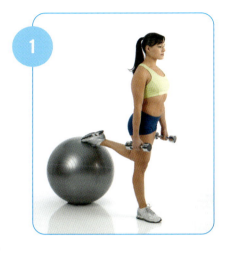

- Stand with the ball on the floor behind you.

- Place one foot on top of the ball and position the other out in front on the floor.

- Hold a dumbbell in each hand. Put your weight on the leg out in front.

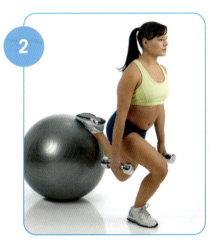

- Lower your body until your back shin touches the ball.

- Keep your back in a neutral position.

- Push through the front foot to return to the starting position.

Intensity

Weight Loss	Toning
3 SETS	3 SETS
15 REPS	8 REPS
30-SECOND REST	30-SECOND REST
BETWEEN SETS	BETWEEN SETS

HINTS

The position of your back is very important in squatting exercises. Always maintain a neutral spine. Don't round your lower back or overarch it. • Keep your head up and look straight ahead. • Place your body weight on your front foot, not on the back foot.

WORKOUT 3: Wall Push-Up

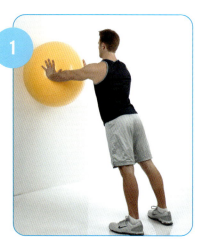

- Stand with your feet hip-width apart facing a wall, holding the ball against the wall. Position your hands on the ball at chest height with your arms fully extended.

- Shift your body weight against the ball.

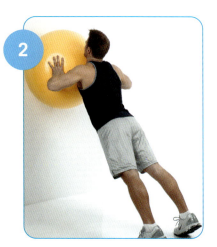

- Lower your body toward the ball, bending at the elbow until your chest touches the ball.

- Push back up to the starting position.

Intensity

Weight Loss	Toning
3 SETS	3 SETS
15 REPS	8 REPS
30-SECOND REST	30-SECOND REST
BETWEEN SETS	BETWEEN SETS

HINTS

Keep your back straight by contracting your core muscles. Do not round your lower back. • Move all the way up and all the way down, until your chest is nearly touching the ball.

WORKOUT 3: Single-Arm Rear Delt Row

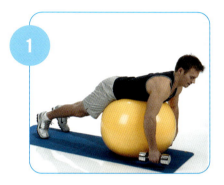

- Lie facedown with the ball under your mid-abdomen and your legs stretched out behind you.

- Hold a dumbbell in one hand with your elbow slightly bent, and your palm facing in.

- Place your other hand on the side of the ball.

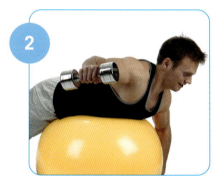

- Lift the dumbbell up and out to the side until it reaches shoulder level.

- Keep your arm straight throughout the exercise, and do not round your upper back.

Intensity

Weight Loss	Toning
3 SETS	3 SETS
15 REPS	8 REPS
30-SECOND REST	30-SECOND REST
BETWEEN SETS	BETWEEN SETS

HINTS

Start with your feet shoulder-width apart. To make it more challenging, bring your feet closer together. • Draw your arm up and out to the side, pulling your shoulder blade to the center of your back at the top position. • Look down at the floor to keep your head in line with your spine. Do not raise your head as you raise the dumbbell.

WORKOUT 3: Dead Lift with Ball to Overhead

1

• Start in a squat position with your feet flat on the floor, your head up, and your back in a neutral position.

• Hold the ball on the floor in front of you.

2

• Stand up and raise the ball overhead with your arms fully extended.

• Lower yourself into a squatting position with the ball on the floor in front of you.

Intensity

Weight Loss	Toning
3 SETS	3 SETS
15 REPS	8 REPS
30-SECOND REST	30-SECOND REST
BETWEEN SETS	BETWEEN SETS

HINTS

Always check your back position in squatting exercises. Always maintain a neutral position. Do not round the lower back or overarch it. • *Keep your head up, looking straight ahead, and your shoulders back.*

WORKOUT 3: Kneeling Lateral Raise

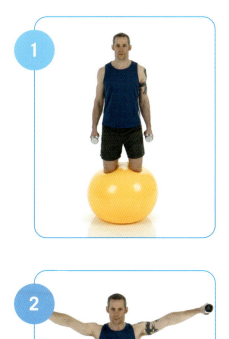

- Kneel upright on the ball, holding a dumbbell in each hand with your palms facing in, and your arms extended by your sides.

- Raise both dumbbells up and out to just above shoulder level, keeping your arms straight.

- Lower the dumbbells to your starting position.

Intensity

Weight Loss	Toning
3 SETS	3 SETS
15 REPS	8 REPS
30-SECOND REST	30-SECOND REST
BETWEEN SETS	BETWEEN SETS

HINTS

Practice kneeling on the ball and become confident before attempting any exercise with weights. • Avoid jerky movements. • Bend your elbows slightly to reduce stress on your shoulder joints.

WORKOUT 3: Chest Fly

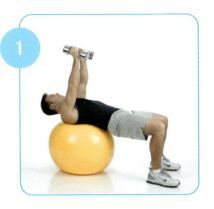

1

- Lie over the ball in a reverse bridge position, centering the ball between your shoulder blades.

- Keep your hips level with your shoulders.

- Hold a dumbbell in each hand, with your arms fully extended overhead, and your palms facing in.

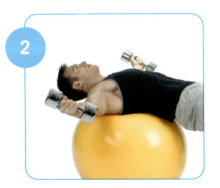

2

- Lower the dumbbells to the sides and down to shoulder level.

- Return to your starting position, extending your arms fully overhead.

- Keep a slight bend in your elbows throughout the exercise.

Intensity

Weight Loss	Toning
3 SETS	3 SETS
15 REPS	8 REPS
30-SECOND REST	30-SECOND REST
BETWEEN SETS	BETWEEN SETS

HINTS

Keep your hips in line with your shoulders. Do not let them sag or dip. This requires you to contract your abdominal and core muscles. • Bend your elbows slightly to reduce stress on the shoulder joint. • Start with your feet shoulder-width apart. To make it more challenging, bring your feet closer together.

WORKOUT 3: **Wall Squat with Bicep Curl**

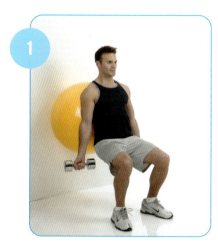

- Stand holding the ball against a wall at your lower-back level.

- Place your feet ahead of the ball, hip-width apart.

- Hold a dumbbell in each hand.

- Lower your body toward the floor, pushing slightly against the ball.

- Stop when your thighs are parallel to the floor.

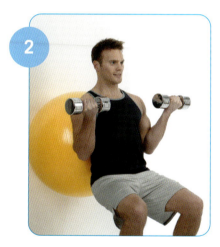

- Holding this squat position, lift the dumbbells up in front to shoulder level, bending your elbows.

- Lower the dumbbells to the starting position at your sides.

Intensity

Weight Loss	Toning
3 SETS	**3 SETS**
15 REPS	**8 REPS**
30-SECOND REST	**30-SECOND REST**
BETWEEN SETS	**BETWEEN SETS**

HINTS

Keep your head up and look straight ahead. Do not look down at the floor or your feet. • Keep your feet flat on the floor with your heels down, as you move the dumbbells up and down. • Keep pushing back against the ball throughout the exercise.

WORKOUT 3: Dips with Hands on ball

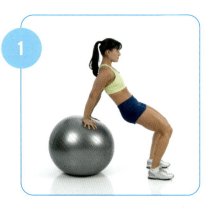

- With the ball behind you, place your hands on top of it with your arms straight and feet flat on the floor in front of you.

- Keep your knees slightly bent.

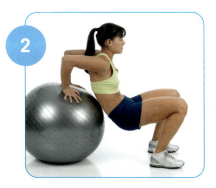

- Lower your body toward the floor by bending your elbows and dropping until your lower back touches the ball.

- Push up against the ball until your arms are straight again in the starting position.

- Keep your feet flat on the floor throughout the exercise.

Intensity

Weight Loss	Toning
3 SETS	**3 SETS**
15 REPS	**8 REPS**
30-SECOND REST	**30-SECOND REST**
BETWEEN SETS	**BETWEEN SETS**

HINTS

Position the ball against a wall to prevent it from moving around. • Do not sit on the ball in the down position; your lower back should barely touch the ball. • To increase the difficulty, straighten your legs and place your heels on the floor. • Keep your head up and look straight ahead.

WORKOUT 3: Pike

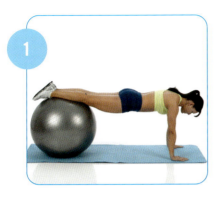

- Start with your hands on the mat directly under your shoulders with your arms fully extended and your shins on the ball.

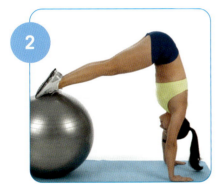

- Drag the ball toward your body, lifting your hips, keeping your legs straight.

- Finish with your feet on the ball.

- Return to the starting position by pushing the ball back out.

Intensity

Weight Loss	Toning
3 SETS	3 SETS
15 REPS	8 REPS
30-SECOND REST	30-SECOND REST
BETWEEN SETS	BETWEEN SETS

HINTS

Keep your hips in line with your shoulders. Do not let them sag or dip. This requires you to contract your abdominal and core muscles throughout the exercise. • Keep your hands under your shoulders in both the starting and top positions. • Start looking down at the floor, and then looking back at the ball, to maintain a neutral spine.

WORKOUT 3: Back Extension with Rotation

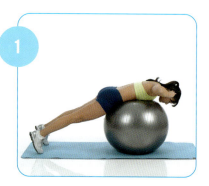

1

- Lie facedown with your chest on the ball with your hands at the sides of your head and your legs extended.

- Let your head and shoulders drape over the ball.

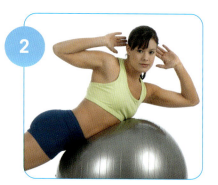

2

- Lift your chest up off the ball, extending through your back, and rotate your upper body to one side.

- Keep your hands at the sides of your head, and return to the starting position with your chest on the ball.

Intensity

Weight Loss	Toning
3 SETS	**3 SETS**
15 REPS	**8 REPS**
30-SECOND REST	**30-SECOND REST**
BETWEEN SETS	**BETWEEN SETS**

HINTS

Lift just your head and shoulders, not your whole upper body. • Keep your shoulders aligned. Do not allow your upper body to fall forward. • Do not overarch your lower back. • Push your toes into the floor to help stabilize you and prevent slipping.

WORKOUT 3: Bridge Shoulder Rolls

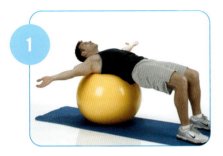

- Lie over the ball with your back in a reverse bridge position and the ball centered between your shoulder blades.

- Keep your hips level with your shoulders.

- Stretch your arms out to the sides holding them up at shoulder level.

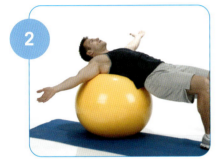

- Roll your upper body across the ball to one side, using your feet to move you.

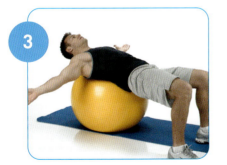

- Roll back to the center, and then to the other side, moving completely across your shoulders.

Intensity

Weight Loss	Toning
3 SETS	**3 SETS**
15 REPS	**8 REPS**
30-SECOND REST	**30-SECOND REST**
BETWEEN SETS	**BETWEEN SETS**

HINTS

Start by taking small steps with your feet. Take bigger steps once you are used to the exercise. • Keep your hips in line with your shoulders. Do not let them sag or dip. This requires you to contract your abdominal and core muscles.

WORKOUT 3: Lower Body Twist

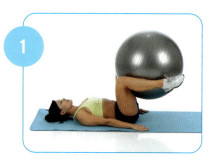

1

- Lie with your back on the mat, your knees bent, and the ball between your feet, off the floor.

- Place your hands at your sides.

2

- Rotate your lower body to one side until that knee touches the floor, still holding the ball between your feet.

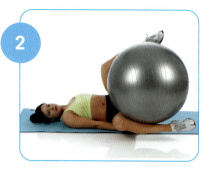

3

- Rotate 180 degrees to the other side, and repeat, touching the floor with your other knee.

Intensity

Weight Loss	Toning
3 SETS	3 SETS
15 REPS	8 REPS
30-SECOND REST	30-SECOND REST
BETWEEN SETS	BETWEEN SETS

HINTS

Keep your shoulders and upper back flat on the mat throughout the exercise. • Twist through your midsection, using your abdominal muscles.

WORKOUT 3: Standing Hamstring Stretch

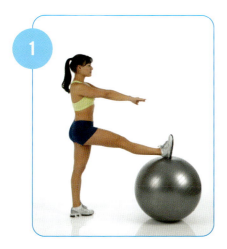

- Stand with one heel set on the ball in front of you.

- Stretch your arms out in front of you and gently lean forward at the waist, moving your hands toward your foot.

Intensity

HOLD FOR 10 SECONDS
REPEAT 3 TIMES WITH EACH LEG

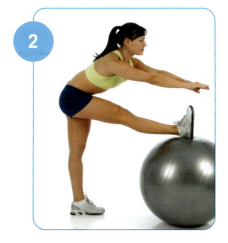

WORKOUT 3: Hip Flexor Stretch

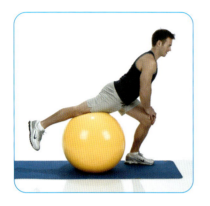

- Stand over the ball with one leg in front and the other behind you.

- Shift your weight forward, opening the back hip joint.

Intensity

HOLD FOR 10 SECONDS
REPEAT 3 TIMES WITH EACH LEG

WORKOUT 3: Lying Hip Abductor Stretch

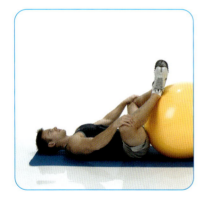

- Lie with your back on the mat and the ball in front of you.

- Position your ankles on the ball with your heels together.

- Gently push your knees away from your body.

Intensity

HOLD FOR 10 SECONDS
REPEAT 3 TIMES

WORKOUT 3: One-Sided Chest Stretch

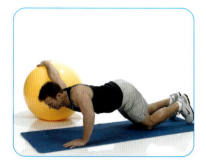

- Kneel on all fours with the ball at one side of you.
- Place your hand on top of the ball with your arm extended.
- Lower your body into a stretch across your upper chest.

Intensity

HOLD FOR 10 SECONDS
REPEAT 3 TIMES WITH EACH ARM

WORKOUT 3: Lateral Stretch

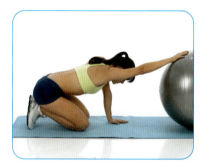

- Kneel on the floor with one hand on top of the ball, at arm's length.
- Keep your head down and look at the floor. Sit back on your heels.
- Lower your shoulder toward the floor until you feel a stretch along the side of your back.

Intensity

HOLD FOR 10 SECONDS
REPEAT 3 TIMES WITH EACH ARM

WORKOUT 4: Step-Up with Ball Overhead

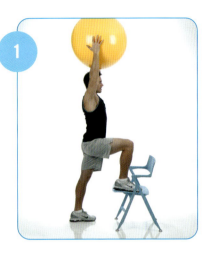

- Start with your arms fully extended overhead, holding the ball in your hands.

- Place one foot on a chair. Keep the other flat on the floor.

- Lean forward, shifting your body weight to the foot on the chair.

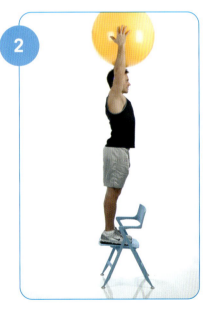

- Push down on your front foot and step up onto the chair.

- Keep the ball overhead with your arms fully extended throughout.

Intensity

Weight Loss	Toning
3 SETS	3 SETS
15 REPS	8 REPS
30-SECOND REST	30-SECOND REST
BETWEEN SETS	BETWEEN SETS

HINTS

Keep your head up and look straight ahead to help maintain a neutral spine. • Put your body weight on the foot on the chair, not on your back foot. • Try not to push off using your back foot. Use the front foot to do the work.

WORKOUT 4: Bridge Bench Press

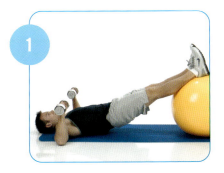

- Lie on your back on the mat with your heels positioned on the ball.

- Raise your hips off the mat by contracting your abdominals, and hold this position throughout the exercise.

- Hold a dumbbell in each hand with your elbows bent and your upper arms on the mat.

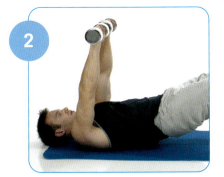

- Lift the dumbbells until your arms are straight.

- Lower the dumbbells by bending your elbows to return to the starting position.

- Lower until your upper arms touch the mat, still holding your hips up and off the mat.

Intensity

Weight Loss	Toning
3 SETS	3 SETS
15 REPS	8 REPS
30-SECOND REST	30-SECOND REST
BETWEEN SETS	BETWEEN SETS

HINTS

Keep your core and abdominal muscles contracted to maintain a neutral spine. • Your head, upper back, and shoulders should contact the mat only at the top position. • Lower the dumbbells until your elbows touch the floor, keeping your forearms vertical.

WORKOUT 4: Reciprocal Wide Row

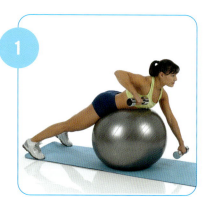

1

- Lie facedown with the ball under your mid-abdomen and your legs stretched out behind you.

- Hold a dumbbell in each hand, one at shoulder level, the other with your arm extended toward the floor.

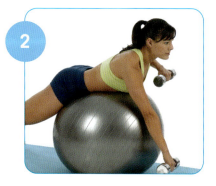

2

- Lift one dumbbell, drawing your shoulder blade in and bending your elbow out. At the same time lower the other dumbbell to the floor in a reciprocal motion.

- Alternate sides, making sure to go all the way down until one dumbbell is nearly at floor level and the other is at shoulder level.

Intensity

Weight Loss	Toning
3 SETS	3 SETS
15 REPS	8 REPS
30-SECOND REST	30-SECOND REST
BETWEEN SETS	BETWEEN SETS

HINTS

Start with your feet shoulder-width apart. To make it more challenging, bring your feet closer together. • *Draw your elbows up and out at your sides, not in close.* • *Look down at the floor to keep your head aligned with your spine. Do not raise your head as you lift the dumbbells.*

WORKOUT 4: **Wall Squat**

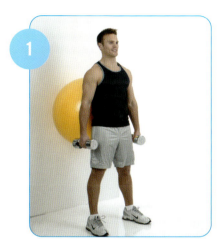

- Stand, holding the ball against a wall at your lower-back level.

- Place your feet ahead of the ball, hip-width apart with your legs straight.

- Hold a dumbbell in each hand.

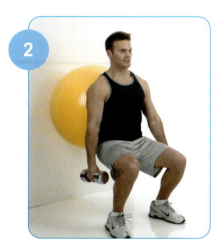

- Lower your body toward the floor, pushing back slightly against the ball.

- Stop when your thighs are parallel to the floor.

- Push through your feet to return to the starting position.

Intensity

Weight Loss	Toning
3 SETS	**3 SETS**
15 REPS	**8 REPS**
30-SECOND REST	**30-SECOND REST**
BETWEEN SETS	**BETWEEN SETS**

HINTS

*Keep your head up and look straight ahead during the exercise. Do not look down at the floor or your feet. •
Keep your feet flat on the floor with your heels down as you move up and down. • Push against the ball
throughout the exercise.*

WORKOUT 4: Kneeling Front Raise

1 • Kneel upright on the ball, holding a dumbbell in each hand with your palms facing down and your arms extended by your sides.

2 • Lift the dumbbells in front to just above shoulder level, keeping your arms straight.

• Lower the dumbbells to the starting position at your sides.

Intensity

Weight Loss	Toning
3 SETS	3 SETS
15 REPS	8 REPS
30-SECOND REST	30-SECOND REST
BETWEEN SETS	BETWEEN SETS

HINTS

Practice kneeling on the ball before attempting any exercise with weights. • Avoid jerky movements. • Bend your elbows slightly to reduce stress on your shoulder joints.

WORKOUT 4: Walk Out

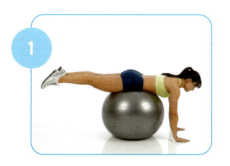

1

- Start with your hands on the mat directly under your shoulders with your arms fully extended and the ball under your abdomen.

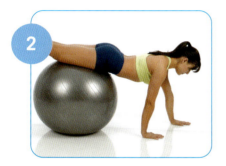

2

- Lift one hand and move it forward. Follow with the other hand.

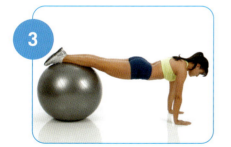

3

- Continue walking your hands forward as you move out until the ball is under your feet.

- Reverse direction and walk your hands back to your starting position.

Intensity

Weight Loss	Toning
3 SETS	**3 SETS**
15 REPS	**8 REPS**
30-SECOND REST	**30-SECOND REST**
BETWEEN SETS	**BETWEEN SETS**

HINTS

Start by taking small steps with your hands. Increase the length of the steps when you are comfortable with the exercise. • Look down at the floor to maintain a neutral spine. Do not raise your head as you move.

WORKOUT 4: Kneeling Hammer Curl

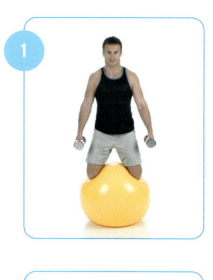

• Kneel upright on the ball, holding a dumbbell in each hand with your palms facing in, and your arms extended along your sides.

• Lift the dumbbells in front to shoulder level, bending your elbows, with your palms facing in.

• Return the dumbbells to your starting position.

Intensity

Weight Loss	Toning
3 SETS	3 SETS
15 REPS	8 REPS
30-SECOND REST	30-SECOND REST
BETWEEN SETS	BETWEEN SETS

HINTS

Practice kneeling on the ball before attempting any exercise using weights. • Keep your back upright by contracting your core muscles. Do not round your lower back. • Complete the full range of motion, from arms fully extended, to dumbbells at shoulder level, and back again.

WORKOUT 4: Kneeling Triceps Extension

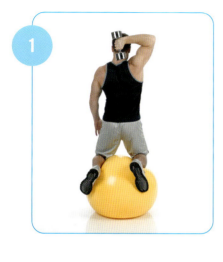

- Kneel upright on the ball.
- Hold a dumbbell in one hand behind your head with your elbow bent.

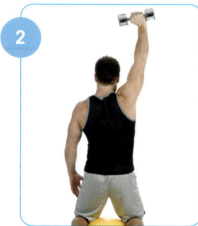

- Lift the dumbbell by extending your elbow and straightening your arm directly overhead.
- Lower the dumbbell to the starting position behind your head.

Intensity

Weight Loss	Toning
3 SETS	3 SETS
15 REPS	8 REPS
30-SECOND REST BETWEEN SETS	30-SECOND REST BETWEEN SETS

HINTS

Practice kneeling on the ball before attempting any exercise with weights. • Be careful not to hit the back of your head with the dumbbell as you lift and lower it. • Do not allow your upper arm to move. Keep your shoulder steady; all movement should occur at your elbow.

WORKOUT 4: **Single-Arm Chest Fly**

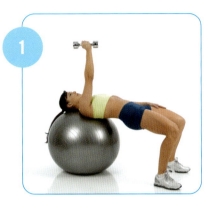

1

- Lie over the ball with your back in a reverse bridge position, centering the ball between your shoulder blades.

- Keep your hips level with your shoulders.

- Hold a dumbbell in one hand with your arm fully extended overhead and your palm facing in. Keep the other arm by your side.

2

- Lower the dumbbell to the side and down to shoulder level.

- Return to your starting position, with your arm fully extended overhead.

- Keep a slight bend in your elbow throughout the exercise.

Intensity

Weight Loss	Toning
3 SETS	**3 SETS**
15 REPS	**8 REPS**
30-SECOND REST	**30-SECOND REST**
BETWEEN SETS	**BETWEEN SETS**

HINTS

Keep your hips in line with your shoulders. Do not let them sag or dip. This requires you to contract your abdominal and core muscles. • Bend your elbow slightly to reduce stress on your shoulder joint. • Start with your feet shoulder-width apart. To make it more challenging, move them closer together.

WORKOUT 4: Seated Twisting Curl on Single Leg

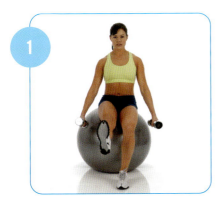

• Sit upright on the ball with one foot flat on the floor and the other leg extended in front.

• Hold a dumbbell in each hand with your palms facing in and your arms extended along your sides.

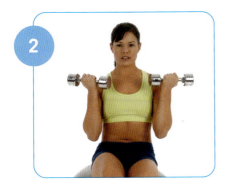

• Lift the dumbbells to shoulder level in front, bending your elbows and twisting your wrists.

• Lower the dumbbells to your starting position.

Intensity

Weight Loss	Toning
3 SETS	3 SETS
15 REPS	8 REPS
30-SECOND REST	30-SECOND REST
BETWEEN SETS	BETWEEN SETS

HINTS

Keep your back upright by contracting your core muscles. Keep your lower back straight. • *Complete the full range of motion, from arms fully extended, to dumbbells at shoulder level, and back again.*

WORKOUT 4: Kneeling Reciprocal Lateral Raise

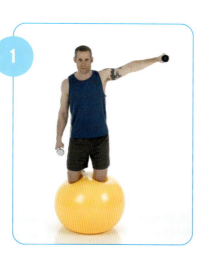

- Kneel upright on the ball, holding a dumbbell in each hand with palms facing in.

- Start with one dumbbell at shoulder height with your arm straight and the other extended along your side.

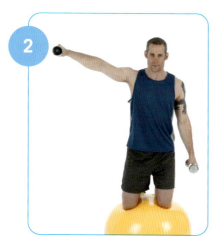

- Raise that dumbbell up and out to just above shoulder level, while lowering the other to your side in a reciprocal motion. Keep both arms straight.

Intensity

Weight Loss	Toning
3 SETS	3 SETS
15 REPS	8 REPS
30-SECOND REST	30-SECOND REST
BETWEEN SETS	BETWEEN SETS

HINTS

Practice kneeling on the ball before attempting any exercise with weights. • Avoid jerky movements. • Bend the elbows slightly to reduce stress on your shoulder joints.

WORKOUT 4: Tuck with One Leg Extended

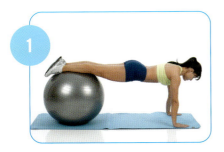

- Start with your hands on the mat directly under your shoulders with your arms fully extended and your shins on the ball.

- Drag the ball toward your hands by bending your knees and bringing them to your chest.

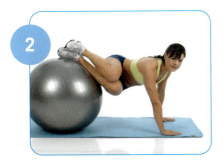

- Rotate your lower body to one side, pulling your knees up and to the side.

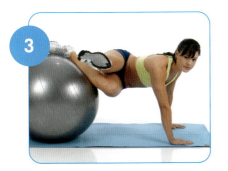

- Extend the top leg out straight.

- Return to the starting position by extending your knees and straightening your legs, pushing the ball out.

- Repeat the exercise, rotating to the other side.

Intensity

Weight Loss	Toning
3 SETS	3 SETS
15 REPS	8 REPS
30-SECOND REST	30-SECOND REST
BETWEEN SETS	BETWEEN SETS

HINTS

Keep your hips in line with your shoulders. Contract your abdominal and core muscles so your hips will not dip. • Look down at the floor to maintain a neutral spin until you rotate, then turn your head to the side.

WORKOUT 4: Weighted Back Extension

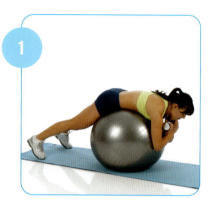

- Lie facedown with your chest on the ball and your legs extended.

- Hold one dumbbell with both hands under your chin, and let your head and shoulders drape over the ball.

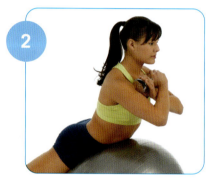

- Lift your chest off the ball, extending through your back with the dumbbell held under your chin.

- Lower your upper body by flexing at the midsection, returning to the starting position.

Intensity

Weight Loss	Toning
3 SETS	**3 SETS**
15 REPS	**8 REPS**
30-SECOND REST	**30-SECOND REST**
BETWEEN SETS	**BETWEEN SETS**

HINTS

Lift only your head and shoulders, not your whole upper body. • Keep your upper body straight at the top of the movement. • Do not overarch your lower back. • Push your toes into the floor to help keep you stable and prevent slipping.

WORKOUT 4: **Wood Chops**

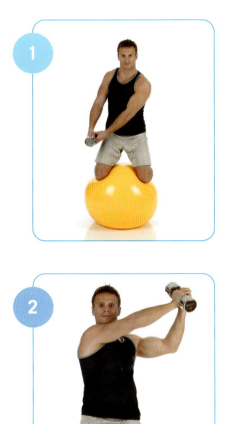

1

- Kneel on the ball, holding one dumbbell with both hands.

- Start with the dumbbell down and to one side.

2

- Raise the dumbbell up, across your body, and over the opposite shoulder.

- Lower the dumbbell down and across your body to the starting position.

Intensity

Weight Loss	Toning
3 SETS	3 SETS
15 REPS	8 REPS
30-SECOND REST	30-SECOND REST
BETWEEN SETS	BETWEEN SETS

HINTS

Practice kneeling on the ball before attempting any exercise with weights. • Avoid jerky movements. • Follow the pattern of chopping a tree, bringing the dumbbell up and over one shoulder, then back down and across the body to the opposite side.

WORKOUT 4: Crunch with Rotation

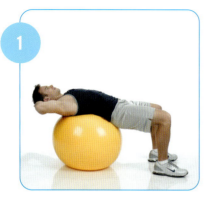

1

- Lie on your back over the ball in a reverse bridge position. Center the ball in your mid-back.

- Keep your head and neck off the ball and your feet flat on the floor.

- Place your hands at the sides of your head.

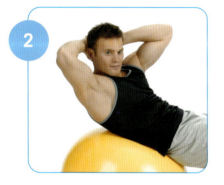

2

- Lift your head and shoulders up and away from the ball and twist to one side, contracting your abdominals and twisting through your midsection.

- Twist back to the center and roll your upper body back over the ball, returning to the starting position.

Intensity

Weight Loss	Toning
3 SETS	3 SETS
15 REPS	8 REPS
30-SECOND REST	30-SECOND REST
BETWEEN SETS	BETWEEN SETS

HINTS

Control the movement through your midsection, and avoid jerky movements. • Do not use your hands to pull your head and neck up. • Start with your feet shoulder-width apart. To make it more challenging, bring your feet closer together.

WORKOUT 4: Lying Hamstring Stretch

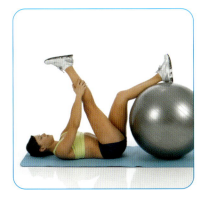

- Lie on your back on the mat. Place one leg on the ball with your knee bent.

- Keep the other leg straight, and clasp your hands behind your calf.

- Slowly pull the straight leg toward your head.

Intensity

HOLD FOR 10 SECONDS
REPEAT 3 TIMES WITH EACH LEG

WORKOUT 4: Glute Stretch

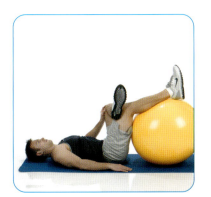

- Lie with your back on the mat. Position one leg on the ball with your knee bent.

- Place the other foot on the bent knee. Use it to gently push the outside knee away from you.

Intensity

HOLD FOR 10 SECONDS
REPEAT 3 TIMES WITH EACH LEG

WORKOUT 4: Standing Hip Abductor Stretch

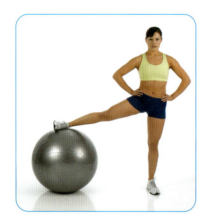

- Stand with the inside ankle of one leg placed on the ball.

- Slowly lower your body, stretching the inside of the leg on the ball.

Intensity

HOLD FOR 10 SECONDS
REPEAT 3 TIMES WITH EACH LEG

WORKOUT 4: Lateral Spine Flexion Stretch

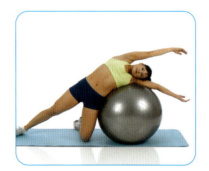

- Kneel beside the ball with your arms extended overhead.

- Lean over the ball as you extend your far leg straight.

Intensity

HOLD FOR 10 SECONDS
REPEAT 3 TIMES ON EACH SIDE

WORKOUT 4: Triceps Stretch

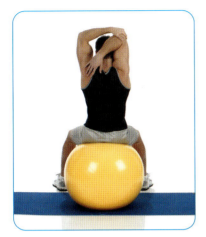

- Sit upright on the ball holding one arm bent at the elbow, behind your head.

- Place the other hand on the bent elbow and slowly pull it across to the middle of your back.

Intensity

HOLD FOR 10 SECONDS
REPEAT 3 TIMES WITH EACH ARM

Index